The Boxing Debate

British Medical Association

June 1993

A publication from the BMA Scientific Department:

Chairman, Board of Science and Education:	Professor J B L Howell
Project Director:	Dr Fleur Fisher
Editor:	David R Morgan
Contributing Authors:	Mr J Brice
	Dr J Cundy
	Dr L D Kartsounis
	Mr J Keast-Butler
	Dr G Roberts
	Sallie Robins
	Dr A Valentine
Editorial secretariat and design:	Hilary Glanville
	Sarah Mars
	Lynne Burton

The Association is grateful for help provided by many individuals and organisations in the preparation of this document. In particular we are pleased to acknowledge the specialist guidance provided by: the Craft Committees of the BMA, Dr C J Bruton, Dr C J Earl, Dr H Grant, Professor B Jennett.

British Library Cataloguing in Publication Data:

British Medical Association (Board of Science and Education)

THE BOXING DEBATE

ISBN 0 7279 0816 2

First published in 1993 by: British Medical Association
Tavistock Square
London WC1H 9JP

Printed by The Chameleon Press Limited, London

Table of Contents

Table of Contents

Legends for pictures

from dementia pugilistica). The boxers' brains are smaller than normal with loss of the surface grey matter and inner white matter. The fluidfilled central cavities are larger than normal, but smaller than those in patient B who had Alzheimer's Disease. The central septum in the boxers' brains are widely separated and torn. This is in marked contrast to the normal septum in A and the narrow stretched septum in B. Location: Page 19

Figure 8   High power view of the septum in boxer's brain, 7C. The 2 leaves of the septum (arrowed) are widely separated and torn. Location: Page 21

Figure 9   Traverse cut through the mid brain of an elderly non boxer (A) to compare with B, C & D. The normal darkly pigmented area (substantia nigra) is clearly visible in A. However, B, C & D show marked loss of pigment. The appearances in C & D are typical of those seen in severe cases of Parkinson's Disease. Location: Page 22

Figures 7, 8 and 9 with kind permission of Dr C J Bruton, Medical Research Council, Runwell Hospital, Wickford, Essex.

Figure 10   Structure of the eye in horizontal section. Location: Page 25

Figure 11a Compression of the eye from a blow causes equatorial expansion and traction at the vitreous base. Location: Page 27

Figure 11b Blow causes eye could more directly push back the vitreous base, leading to shearing the the development of retinal tears. Location: Page 28

Figure 12   CT scan of the brain of an elderly ex-boxer suffering from dementia. There is severe atrophy of the cortex and white matter and marked dilation of the ventricles (A). Location: Page 35

Figure 13   CT scan of boxer's brain: white stripe on the left of skull (marked A with dotted line) represents an acute subdural haematoma. Location: Page 36

Figure 14   MRI of normal brain: note small ventricles (arrows A) and absent or narrow subarachnoid space (arrows B). Location: Page 38

Figure 15   MRI following head injury: note large ventricles(A) and generous subarachnoid space (arrows B) indicating atrophy of the cortex. Location: Page 39

Figure 16   The use of headguards protects against superficial injury but cannot eliminate the dangerous accelerating and decelerating forces applied to the head. (Popperfoto) Location: Page 70

Table 4.1   Studies carried out since publication of the 1984 boxing report. Location: Pages 42-43

List of acronyms

ABA	Amateur Boxing Association
AD	Alzheimer's disease
ARM	Annual Representatives' Meeting
BBBC	British Boxing Board of Control
BMJ	British Medical Journal
BMA	British Medical Association
CNS	central nervous system
CSF	cerebrospinal fluid
CSP	cavum septum pellucidum
CT	computed tomography
DP	dementia pugilistica
EEG	electroencephalography
HMPAO	hexamethylpropylene amine oxime
SPECT	single photon emission computed tomography
JAMA	Journal of the American Medical Association
MAO	monoamine oxidase
MRI	magnetic resonance imaging
NABC	National Association of Boys Clubs
OPCS	Office of Population Censuses and Surveys
PET	positron emission tomography
PTA	post traumatic amnesia
RA	retrograde amnesia
SABA	Schools Amateur Boxing Association
WBO	World Boxing Organisation

Glossary

Acute
: Any condition which is sudden, severe and of short duration.

Alzheimer's disease
: A condition resulting in memory failure for recent events and lack of spontaneous activity and initiative. Due to degenerative changes in the brain.

Amygdaloid nucleus
: An almond shaped area of the brain adjoining the hippocampus (qv). It responds to smells and other senses and is important for memories that link sensory and emotional experiences such as fear.

Analysis of covariance
: Statistical technique used to analyse data where there are a wide range of variables used to identify the effect of the variables on results.

Aqueous
: Fluid filling the front chamber of the eye. Similar to blood but under normal circumstances it is entirely without red or white cells and almost entirely devoid of protein.

Arachnoid mater
: A delicate membrane enveloping the brain and spinal cord.

Atrophy
: Wasting of a tissue or organ.

BRITISH MEDICAL ASSOCIATION

Autoregulation	The ability of the circulation in the brain to adjust to influences that may threaten blood flow to the brain, eg inflammation.
Basal ganglia	A poorly understood complex of centres within the cerebral hemispheres (qv) involved in skilled motor responses.
Beta amyloid protein	Protein characteristically found in the brains of individuals suffering from Alzheimer's disease.
Calcarine sulcus	A groove on the inner side of the cerebral hemisphere which marks the site in the cortex concerned with vision.
Capillary permeability	The degree to which fluid can pass through the walls of capillary blood vessels.
Cavum septum pellucidum	Also known as the 'fifth ventricle' of the brain. Fluid filled cavity surrounded by the septum pellucidum. Normally not present in adults as cavity closes in infants shortly after birth. Controversy surrounds whether its presence in adults is indicative of prior head injury.
Cerebellar hemispheres (cerebellum)	A mass of grey and white matter on either side of the centre of the brain concerned with the production of skilled movement mainly of the upper limbs. Liable to damage in its lower portion from blows to the head.
Cerebral hemispheres (cerebrum)	One on either side form the major mass of the brain. They are covered in cortex and control almost all of the higher functions of an individual.
Cerebrospinal fluid	A clear, colourless fluid made in the ventricles of the brain and circulating within the skull and spine, supporting and

protecting the brain. Takes the place of brain that has disappeared following trauma (qv).

Choroid	Lining of the white of the eye.
Chronic	Of long duration; the opposite of acute (qv).
Computed tomography	Method of structural brain imaging using x-rays.
Contusion	A bruise.
Cornea	Disc of clear tissue covering the front of the eye.
Corpus callosum	Structure within the brain co-ordinating the activities of the two sides of the brain.
Cortex	A layer of grey matter containing the cerebral hemispheres. This tissue controls and organises the responses of the individual to the environment. Liable to damage when it comes into contact with the overlying skull.
Dementia Pugilistica	The Punch Drunk syndrome. A progressive neurodegenerative syndrome related to continual minor brain damage with symptoms progressing from mild incoordination to global cognitive decline and parkinsonism.
Dementia	A form of mental disorder in which the cognitive and intellectual functions of the mind are prominently or predominantly affected.
Dura mater	The outermost membrane of the brain that is thick, dense and inelastic. It lines the interior of the skull.

Electroencephalo-graphy	Mechanism of measuring brain function by registering the electric current set up in the cerebral cortex by the action of the brain. Usually refers to brain activity recorded by electrodes placed on the scalp.
Endothelium lining	A cellular covering of cavities in the body.
Falx cerebri	Sickle-shaped fold of dura mater which lies between the two cerebral hemispheres.
Foramen magnum	The opening in the base of the skull through which the brain stem joins the spinal cord.
Fornix	A band of white matter lying within the ventricles connected to the limbic system and hence is concerned with emotional activity.
Frontal lobes	The greater portion of the cerebral hemisphere (qv) lying in the front of the skull. Controls behaviour in all its aspects. Particularly liable to surface damage after a blow on the head.
Fusiform gyrus	A fold of cortex in the temporal lobe. Part of the limbic system concerned with emotional activity. Liable to damage in its anterior portion.
Glaucoma	Raised pressure in the eyeball which can cause progressive loss of vision.
Gliosis	An increase in certain cells of the brain when damage has occurred. Can be regarded as a scar in the brain.
Haemorrhage	A leakage of blood from its vessels.

Hippocampus | A fold of cortex on the inner surface of the temporal lobe. Vital for some forms of learning and memory and liable to damage after head injury. Patients with a damaged hippocampus cannot form memories of new events.

Hydrocephalus | Enlargement of the skull due to an abnormal collection of cerebrospinal fluid around the brain or in the ventricles.

Hypothalamus | A small area of grey matter surrounding the basal ventricular system. Important in the control of basic functions of the body (eg sexual activity).

Inferior cortex of cerebellum | The surface layers of the cerebellum lying in the base of skull above the foramen magnum (qv). Found to be damaged in some ex-boxers' brains.

Internal capsule | A wide band of fibres passing to and from the cortex (qv).

Intracerebral clots | Clots of blood within the brain.

Intracranial pressure | The pressure of the tissues inside the skull.

Iris | Coloured part of the eye.

Lesion | An injury, wound, or morbid structural change in an organ.

Limbic system | The structures within the brain, such as the hippocampus and amygdaloid nucleus, responsible for drives, emotions and behaviour associated with basic survival: pain, pleasure, fear, anger, feeding and sexual feelings.

Magnetic Resonance Imaging	Method of structural brain imaging using radio waves and magnetic fields.
Medial Temporal lobe	The wide surface of the temporal lobe (qv) containing much of the limbic system (emotional brain). Particularly susceptible to damage following a blow to the head.
Morbidity	Disease or ill-health.
Mortality	Death.
Neuropathologist	A medical practitioner, usually a trained pathologist, who specialises in the diagnosis of diseases of the nervous system through laboratory work and the study of bodies after death (autopsy).
Neuropsychometric testing	Tests used to identify the behavioral expression of brain dysfunction.
Neuroscientist	General term for a specialist in the science of the nervous system (eg a neurosurgeon).
Neurosurgeon	A medical practitioner, usually skilled in general surgery, who specialises in operating on diseases of the nervous system and looks after patients suffering from severe head injury.
Ora Serrata	Jagged edge of the retina.
Orbit	The eye socket.

Parahippocampal gyrus Structure within the limbic system of the brain. Part of the medial temporal lobe (qv).

Parenchymal damage Damage to the essential active cells of an organ as distinguished from vascular and connective tissue.

Parkinson's disease A condition of late middle life characterised by a mask-like face, rigidity of the limbs with tremor of the hands and general clumsiness of muscular movements due to degenerative changes in the brain.

Periventricular tissues Tissues surrounding the ventricles (qv) of the brain.

Pigment epithelium Layer of cells within the choroid of the eye.

Positron emission computed tomography Method of detecting the decay of radionuclides introduced into the brain to assess brain function.

Hexamethypropylene amine oxime Compound used in conjunction with positron emission computed tomography. Its distribution in the brain is determined by blood flow and it can therefore be used to detect defects in cerebral blood flow.

Punch Drunk syndrome Dementia Pugilistica. A progressive neurodegenerative syndrome related to continual minor brain damage with symptoms progressing from mild incoordination to global cognitive decline and parkinsonism.

Purkinje Cells Large nerve cells in the cerebellar cortex involved in the production of fine, graceful movements.

Retina	The innermost coat of the eyeball, responsible for channelling visual information to the optic nerve.
Sclera	White of the eye.
Septum pellucidum	A thin two layered partition which separates the right from the left lateral ventricle of the brain. Function unknown. Frequently found to be torn when the brains of ex-boxers have been examined.
Spinal Cord	A long cylindrical mass of grey and white matter running in the spinal canal. It has many functions, one of which is to transmit messages from the brain to the periphery of the body.
Subarachnoid space	Space between the arachnoid mater and adjacent tissue, filled with cerebrospinal fluid. Often enlarged in chronic brain injury.
Subdural haematoma	An accumulation of blood plasma or clot beneath the dura mater, displacing the brain.
Substantia nigra	A collection of black coloured cells on either side of the upper brain stem. Degeneration of this area of the brain is associated with the Parkinson-like symptoms seen in some ex-boxers.
Temporal lobes	Two large portions of the cerebral hemisphere lying beneath the temple and above the ear. Major functions are those of memory and emotional activity. Liable to surface damage in head injury.
Traction	The act of pulling.

Thalamus	A large, egg-shaped structure located above the midbrain, consisting of two masses of grey matter covered by a thin layer of white matter, lying deeply in each cerebral hemisphere. Directs messages about sight, hearing, taste and touch and assists in planning and controlling movements.
Trauma	A wound or injury.
Upper brain stem	A complex structure lying below the thalamus (qv) transmitting impulses from above and below. One of the major centres of consciousness and control of the eyes.
Ventricle	A small pouch or cavity eg the cavities of the brain.
Vitreous	Tissue filling the rear chamber of the eye, consists almost entirely of intercellular glue with a little additional supportive tissue.
White matter	Tissues composed largely of the tentacles (axons) of the brain cells which connect one brain cell with another. May be stretched and torn in injury. Not capable of effective functional repair.

Introduction

The British Medical Association (BMA) has become a leading authority on the hazards of boxing since 1982 when a resolution passed at the Annual Representatives Meeting (ARM) stated, *that in view of the proven ocular and brain damage resulting from professional boxing, the Association should campaign for its abolition.* In response to this resolution the Board of Science and Education of the BMA set up a working party to review the evidence on brain and eye damage as a result of boxing injuries and to publish a report of their findings. In the final report of the working party published in 1984, it was concluded that damage occurred to the eye and brain in both amateur and professional boxers.

Following the widespread publicity given to the BMA report, there appeared to be strong opposition to a total ban from a number of sources. The working party's findings were criticised by the British Boxing Board of Control (BBBC) and others as relating to foreign studies and research undertaken before measures to improve safety had been introduced by the BBBC. In addition, the Amateur Boxing Association (ABA) professed the safety of amateur boxing and the National Association of Boys Clubs (NABC) continued to support amateur boxing within its clubs.

The 1984 report of the Boxing working party continued to be widely discussed both within and outside the profession and a further resolution was passed at the 1987 ARM stating, *that in view of the continuing serious ill effects on the health of boxers, this Meeting requests the BMA to pursue the Government with renewed vigour until there is a ban on boxing, and until such time as this is achieved, believes that television coverage should include a statement of the damage which may result from boxing.*

The Board of Science and Education, individual members of the BMA, and the press and parliamentary department of the BMA, have continued over the years to promulgate the evidence for harm caused by boxing. The BMA has provided speakers at the Cambridge Union, technical colleges, the annual meeting of the Amateur Boxing Association doctors, and many local BMA divisions. In 1991 Lord Taylor of Gryfe presented a bill in the House of Lords to abolish "boxing for profit". This bill was lost by only two votes and the arguments presented by the BMA were well received and widely reported.

Since publication of the report on boxing in 1984 there have been developments within the control of boxing and in attitudes to boxing, as well as advances in the medical field enabling the early detection of damage to the brain due to head injury. The Board of Science and Education therefore set up a boxing steering group to review the evidence on boxing injuries published in the past seven years. This initiative was supported by the 1992 ARM of the BMA where two further resolutions on boxing were passed stating, *that the forthcoming publication of the revised report on boxing be welcomed* and *that this meeting calls for a total ban on amateur and professional boxing in the UK.* The ARM also passed a policy on boxing among children stating, *that this meeting believes that as the next stage of our campaign against boxing we should seek a ban on children below the age of consent from boxing.* These policies reaffirm the BMA's position in opposing both amateur and professional boxing because of the chronic and acute brain injuries that arise.

Scope of the report

This report reviews the existing evidence on injuries related to boxing and considers the mechanisms by which injuries occur and the available techniques for detecting such injuries.

Chapter One provides a brief history of boxing. The development of boxing into its current form is outlined to provide a backdrop to the subsequent discussion of the dangers associated with boxing contests. Chapter Two analyses the mechanisms by which injury occurs to the brain and to the eye in boxing. The type of blows that occur during a boxing bout are outlined to reveal how they may result in both acute and chronic damage.

Chapter Three summarises the available techniques for detecting brain injury in boxers. Imaging and non imaging techniques are detailed as well as those techniques enabling examination of the functioning of the brain.

Chapter Four examines the medical evidence for injuries occurring in boxing, published since the 1984 report. The available evidence is reviewed in relation to the detection techniques employed by research workers and conclusions on the dangers of boxing are drawn from the results.

Chapter Five reviews the debate on boxing. The views of those in favour and against boxing are highlighted alongside information gathered by the BMA during its campaign of the past 10 years. The legal position of boxing is questioned and boxing in the Armed Forces and amongst young children considered.

This report was prepared under the auspices of the Board of Science and Education of the British Medical Association. The members of the Board were as follows:

Sir John Reid	President, BMA
Dr W J Appleyard	Chairman, Representative Body, BMA
Dr J Lee-Potter	Chairman, BMA Council
Dr A Riddell	Treasurer, BMA
Professor J B L Howell	Chairman, Board of Science and Education
Professor J P Payne	Deputy Chairman, Board of Science and Education
Dr J M Cundy	
Dr A Elliott	
Dr R Farrow	
Dr R Gilbert	
Dr L P Grime	
Dr K Hildyard	
Dr A Mitchell	
Dr G M Mitchell	
Col M J G Thomas L/RAMC	
Dr D Ward	

A Steering Group with the following membership was set up in order to provide expert guidance:

Mr J Brice	Consultant Neurosurgeon, Wessex Regional Health Authority/University of Southampton General Hospitals
Dr J Cundy	Member, BMA Board of Science and Education, Consultant Anaesthetist, Lewisham University Hospital
Dr P K P Harvey	Consultant Neurologist, The Royal Free Hospital
Professor J P Payne	Member, BMA Board of Science and Education, Emeritus Professor of Anaesthesia, University of London
Dr G W Roberts	Neuroscientist, Department of Anatomy and Cell Biology, St Mary's Hospital Medical School, Imperial College of Science Technology and Medicine, London

CHAPTER ONE

A Brief History of Boxing

The origins of boxing are lost in the mists of prehistoric time. Accounts of the early days of boxing are, therefore, likely to be based on speculation, rather than evidence. It is probable that early human beings living together in settlements would have settled arguments, on occasion, by an exchange of blows. However, it is equally likely that primitive man would face too many threats to his wellbeing from everyday life to risk injury from such contests arranged in the name of sport or entertainment.

As man became more successful in his competition with natural forces so boxing as a contest began to develop. There is hieroglyphic evidence of boxing in Ethiopia as early as 4000 BC and it spread to Egypt via the Nile Valley. By 1500 BC boxing was practised in Ancient Crete as it followed the spread of the Egyptian civilisation throughout the eastern Mediterranean. Almost a thousand years later in 686 BC boxing was introduced into the Olympic Games in Greece where contestants were induced to perform by the promise of glory and wealth. The unsuccessful combatants were unlikely to enjoy any benefit, however, as contests continued without any rest period, until one boxer was unable to continue to put up a resistance, however weak it might be.

At this time protection of the hands was introduced to enable fighters to land heavier blows. At first fists were bound with soft leather but as the need for more

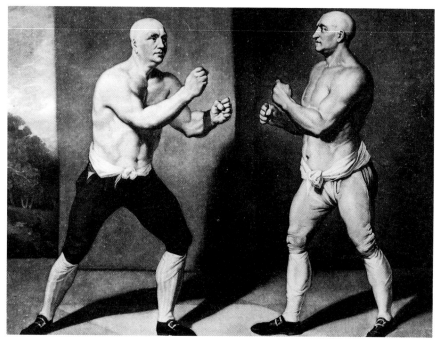

Figure 1:
Boxing in the 18th century: Jack Broughton (left) and James Figg.

spectator excitement developed, the leather became harder and ultimately in the latter days of the Roman Empire the notorious "caestus" appeared. This glove was clearly an effective weapon, as the striking surface was studded with brass or iron knobs. Members of underprivileged ethnic minorities were encouraged to fight using these fearsome weapons until the death of one or other contestant occurred for the entertainment of their wealthy Roman masters. Thereafter, pugilism as entertainment ceased to exist for several centuries. In fact, through the Dark Ages and the Renaissance nothing is recorded of its existence in Europe. During this time, however, Chinese, Japanese and other Eastern nations had developed their own forms of martial art.

In 1681, a formal bout was recorded in the UK and soon thereafter regular contests were held in London. These were the days of prizefighting; the contestants fought without gloves in the beginning of the bare knuckle era. There were no rules and no weight divisions and the contest continued, as in Olympic times, until one man could no longer continue. The bouts were a mixture of boxing and wrestling and it was common to hit a man when he was down. Prizefighting was illegal however, and there are many tales of subterfuges adopted to enable public contests to take place. At Long Reach near Dartford in Kent it is said that contests took place near a public house on the bank of the river Thames and if the forces of the law were spotted approaching across the marshes the spectators and contestants jumped into boats, placed there for this purpose, and rowed across the river to continue in Essex, beyond the reach of the law. It is interesting to note that even in the 1990s the legal status of boxing in Britain remains questionable; it has been suggested that if it can be established that in a boxing contest there is significant danger of permanent injury, then the basis upon which boxing has been held not to be criminal but a lawful sport, "intended to give strength, skill and activity", falls away. This issue is discussed in more detail in the final chapter of this report.

In 1719 James Figg (see Figure 1) opened a school of arms in London's Oxford Road. A year later he fought Ned Sutton, won and became boxing's first modern champion. Thereafter, boxing crossed the Channel into Europe and in 1733 the first international contest took place between an Englishman and an Italian. Following the death of his opponent after a bout Jack Broughton, in 1743, devised a set of rules which remained in force for nearly 100 years (see Figure 2). For this he became known as the "Father of Boxing". Briefly, these rules allowed wrestling holds, although grabbing an opponent "below his waist" was disallowed. The first modern type of boxing glove, known as a "muffler", was introduced and after a man was knocked down he was given 30 seconds rest before continuing or he lost the fight. Furthermore, hitting an opponent on the floor was not allowed.

In 1838, the rules were changed again to what were known as the London Prize Ring Rules. For the first time a ring of ropes 24 feet square was used. A mark was placed in the centre of the ring to which a fighter had to go before being allowed to continue to fight. Kicking, biting, eye gouging, butting and low blows were outlawed. However, due to the continued brawling that took place around the match, boxing still held little appeal for the educated and the wealthy. A completely new set of rules, the Queensbury rules, were therefore set up under the name of the Marquess specifically to attract such audiences and hence more money. All contestants were to wear gloves and to fight for three minute rounds with a rest in between. Wrestling

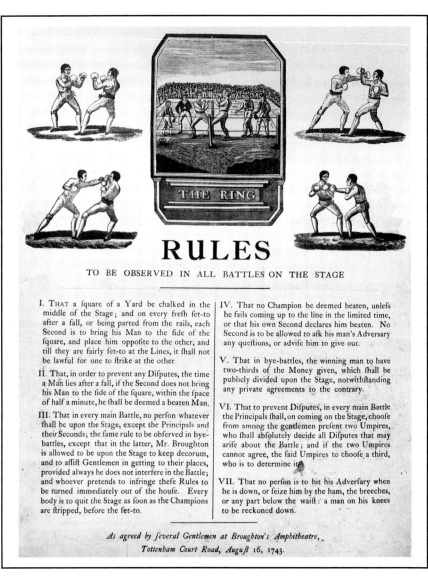

Figure 2
The set of rules drawn up by Jack Broughton in 1743.

was outlawed and the concept of the knock-out was introduced; that is that after being knocked down the boxer had to get up unaided within ten seconds. Weight divisions were also introduced. These rules formed the foundation of modern boxing rules.

Meanwhile boxing had spread to the United States where entrepreneurs realised the enormous profit potential of so-called championship fights. In the present century, boxing has spread to many parts of the world. This has resulted in numerous championships and, although the American National Boxing Association was formed in 1921 to regulate world championships, the world has seen a proliferation of ruling bodies each with their own world champions and there may be three different world champions at any particular weight. Furthermore, the weight divisions have increased so that there are now up to 17 weight divisions whereas

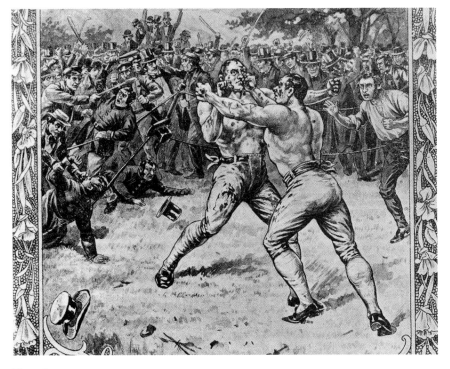

Figure 3
Boxing in the 19th century: second fight between Harry Poulson and Tom Paddock, 16 December 1851.

early on there were only eight. The most important reason for this situation is the rapid increase in media interest which began in the 1920s and took off in immense proportions with the advent of world television. This interest results in enormous amounts of money available to boxers, managers and promoters and their accompanying entourage.

Examination of the lists of world professional champions takes us back to the days of the Roman games. It is clear that the better boxers are once again drawn from underprivileged ethnic minorities. The hopes of status and money, which very few achieve, encourage boxers to contemplate risking their health and lives in a dangerous contest.

The various bodies that have developed in this country to control and organise boxing have done a great deal to make boxing safer for the contestant. The introduction of padded rings with an appropriate number of ropes, the training of referees with the ability to stop fights when one man cannot defend himself, the more precise definition of foul blows and the knock-out, and the introduction of medical supervision of fights have all contributed a great deal to the safety of boxing. Unfortunately at the same time, television interest, with the concentration on the knock-out punch, a punch in which it is certain that brain damage has occurred, has had a reverse effect. Reminiscent of the introduction of the Roman "caestus", this emphasis on the boxer's most dangerous punches removes much of the skill of offensive and defensive boxing, which the points system of scoring — whereby points are awarded for defence and style — was supposed to encourage, and increases the risk of brain damage within the boxing ring. In addition, the variations between different officials awarding points at the same contest leads to the knock-out being the only certain way to win, and implies that extra points are given for brain damage. More recently in Britain, guidelines have been drawn up to improve the care of injured boxers. These may be of some value but only come into effect once brain damage has occurred.

Background material

Encyclopaedia Britannica, Macropaedia: Knowledge in Depth. 1991;**28**:173-175.

Encyclopaedia Britannica, Micropaedia: Ready Reference. 1991;**2**:443-444.

Marrian I. *The Guinness World Championship Boxing Book*. London, Guinness Publishing Ltd, 1990.

CHAPTER TWO

Mechanisms of Injury Sustained During Boxing Contests

This chapter looks at the mechanisms by which blows received in a boxing contest can result in injury to the brain and to the eye. The structure of the brain and eye are outlined and provide the necessary background information to understand the consequences of damage. Appendix four to this report contains a more general overview of the processes that occur in the brain after trauma.

Injury to the brain

Anatomy of a punch

During the course of a boxing match, the contestants receive a variable number of blows to the upper torso, arms and head. These blows land on the target with widely differing degrees of force. The lightest may be a mere flick of a glove and the heaviest, may be as much as half a ton, which has been likened to being hit by a

12 lb padded wooden mallet travelling at 20 miles per hour.[1] A considerable amount of energy is therefore applied to the target area when significant punches hit a boxer. In the case of the torso and arms, the bony structures are covered by skin, fat and well-developed muscles, all of which absorb energy in much the same way as the crumple zone on the front of a car absorbs much of the force of impact in a collision. Although there may be superficial bruising, usually little damage is done to underlying structures. In the case of the head, however, the skin is taught over the underlying skull and its bony projections, such as the eye sockets. There is limited energy absorption and the greater amount of the force of the blow is transmitted directly to the skull and its contents, the brain. Occasionally, over bony projections, especially round the eyes, the skin may split producing the familiar "cut".

Training, experience and skill may enable a boxer to reduce the force received from the blows of their opponent. The boxer learns to move away from the blow, "riding the punch" as it is called, diverting much of the force of the blow so that it glances off the side of the head, forearm or gloves. Strong muscles in the shoulders, upper chest, and neck, may reduce the resulting movement of the head when struck and, as mentioned later, this may reduce the damage to the brain. In spite of all these defensive measures a boxer will receive significant punches in all but the most one-sided contest. Increased and more scientifically based training will increase the weight of the punches delivered by a particular boxer in the same way that modern training improves all athletic performance. The effect of media interest, especially television, is to emphasise the importance of the heavy blow, the knock-out punch. This is exemplified by the regular slow motion analysis of such punches that television provides. Professional boxers may therefore be encouraged to concentrate on heavy punching rather than skilful defence. Such trends and effects nullify the benefits of fitness and training and increase the risk to an individual boxer.

Another factor in the production of brain damage is the unique anatomy of the head and brain. The head is attached to the body by a flexible neck. Heavy blows to the head may produce accelerating and decelerating movements of the head. These movements are momentarily extremely violent, measured on a static target as up to 520 m/s^2 of acceleration.[1] Movement of the head occurs in a variety of planes; for instance, an "upper cut" will tend to produce rotation of the head around a horizontal plane passing across the neck parallel to the shoulders just below the level of the ears. A "swinging hook" or a "cross-counter" punch to the side of the jaw will produce a

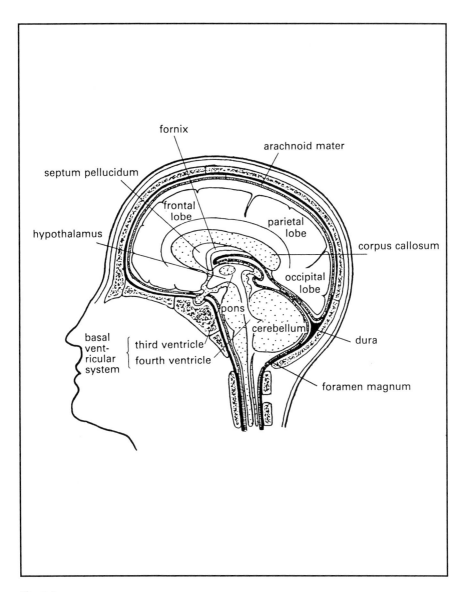

Figure 4
Simplified vertical section of the brain in the midline of the skull.

rotation of the head in a vertical plane passing down through the head and neck behind the ears. This movement is particularly damaging possibly because the neck muscles are at a mechanical disadvantage in preventing rotation in this plane. This rotation is commonly seen in slow motion picture analysis of a knock-out punch and may be recognised by an accompanying spray of sweat and saliva. In this instance the jaw behaves as a long lever applied to the skull and increases the momentum of head movement. It is for this reason that the "point" of the jaw, in boxing parlance, is just to one side or other of the anatomical extremity of the lower jaw. All boxers know that a strong punch landing on this area is likely to lead to a "win by knock-out" because of the brain damage that this movement produces. A short neck and strong muscular development of the shoulder girdle and neck muscles may reduce the speed and force of such rotational movement but only protects the fighter to a limited extent from the effects of the blows delivered. It is these movements of the head in space and in relation to the rest of the boxer's body that give rise to the larger part of brain damage sustained by a boxer.

Structure of the skull and brain

The structure within the human skull also contributes to brain damage. The brain rests inside the skull firmly fixed to the skull base by blood vessels and emerging nerves, including the spinal cord (see Figures 4, 5 and 6). The bulk of the brain (the cerebral and cerebellar hemispheres) is not connected to the skull or its linings except by thin elastic veins and fine strands of arachnoid mater. The cerebral hemispheres and, to a lesser extent, the cerebellar hemispheres are therefore relatively free to move independently of the surrounding skull. Such independent movement depends in part on their respective inertial characteristics. The inner surface of a skull of a muscular young adult male is not smooth and has sharp inward projections. It is tearing of the thin superficial veins and surface damage to the brain as it collides with the skull and its sharp inward projections that give rise to acute subdural haematoma that is responsible for the serious cerebral compression and death that occasionally follows a boxing match.[2,3]

The brain itself is of a firm jelly-like consistency with string-like blood vessels running within its substance. It is not of uniform consistency, the more solid basal ganglia and thalamus being tougher and denser than the surrounding white matter

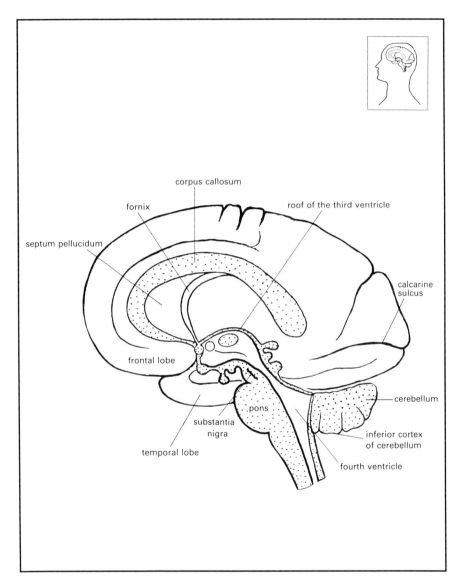

Figure 5
Inside surface of one half of the brain. The upper part of the cerebellum has been 'cut away'.

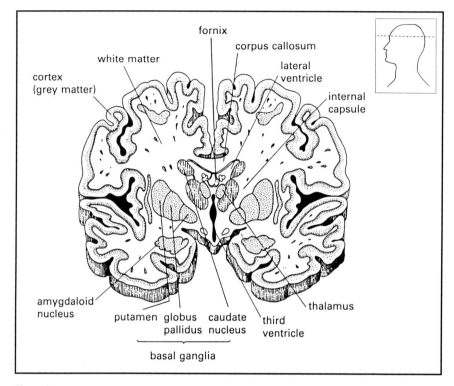

Figure 6
Side-to-side section of the cerebral hemispheres through a line between the two ears.

and cortex. These denser parts of the brain have different inertial characteristics from those of the lighter white matter and to the watery consistency of the cerebral spinal fluid in the ventricles. When the head is struck forcibly and is subject to sharp acceleration followed by a somewhat slower decelerating movement the brain will move at a different rate to the skull. Furthermore, due to the differing inertial characteristics of the different parts of the brain, there will be different rates of movement within the brain itself. This process results in:

(a)   Some surface damage to the cortex, particularly those parts furthest from the point or plane of rotation. In this way maximum damage is likely to occur in the frontal and temporal lobes of the cerebrum and inferior cortex of the cerebellum.

(b)   There will be a "swirling" effect within the brain itself, giving rise to tension between various parts of the brain. This will affect neurological function and, if severe enough, will result in multiple tears of neuronal networks (Strich lesions)[4]. There will also be tension between the brain tissue and contained blood vessels causing further shearing lesions and, in severe cases, bleeding close to the blood vessels.[5,6] Blood flow may be reduced in the affected vessels. These changes are more marked low down in the cerebral hemispheres where there is different mobility of the brain structure, eg, the deep periventricular tissues and substantia nigra in the upper brainstem.

(c)   There will be pressure waves set up within the ventricular system which may explain the high incidence of perforations to the septum pellucidum seen in the brains of former boxers. Such waves of pressure may affect the function of vital centres surrounding the basal ventricular system. There will be similar pressure waves occurring within the brain tissue itself, perhaps less important in boxing injuries than in other more severe blunt injuries. These pressure waves affect the small blood vessels of the brain, causing changes in the endothelial lining and hence, in capillary permeability which adds to the damage to the brain by increasing intracranial pressure and reducing blood flow to the injured areas. These vascular changes can be seen in radioisotope scanning techniques and magnetic resonance scanning techniques, both of which will detect changes in capillary permeability and consequent increase in tissue fluid at the site of injury, as well as changes in local blood flow. (Scanning techniques are reviewed in Chapter Three)

(d)   Rarely, in severe injuries following boxing contests, large intracerebral clots may form. Evidence of acute haemorrhage is frequently seen in the brains of ex-boxers who have died of injuries sustained in the ring. In addition, evidence of minor haemorrhage is frequently seen in the brains of ex-boxers who have died after a long career.[6]

Effects on the boxer

All these complex effects occur at the time of impact of the punch or within a short time thereafter. If severe enough they will cause a deterioration in neurological function. This may show itself to the boxer as a feeling of "grogginess" and a sensation of weakness or paralysis has been recorded by some boxers. The observer may see a weakening of the boxer's legs and there may be a lack of focusing of the eyes. Should these effects not be apparent to the boxer or the referee, further blows of a similar nature may be sustained. Unfortunately, the brain is more susceptible to damage from these subsequent injuries. As a result of increase in tissue fluid the brain may show less tensile strength. The blood vessels may dilate locally and their walls will be more susceptible to rupture. There will be a loss of autoregulation in the damaged blood vessels, that is, their ability to respond to a drop in perfusion pressure may disappear, further threatening the viability of the local tissue. Thus further significant blows are always more dangerous than the initial one. Changes in neurological function affect the ability of the boxer to defend himself or to "ride punches". Subsequent blows may therefore have a much greater effect than the initial one. More severe damage results in a loss of consciousness and the boxer sustains a "knock-out". Perhaps the more fortunate boxer is the one who receives a significant punch early in the fight, is knocked unconscious and spared further punishment. The boxer likely to sustain extensive brain damage is the fighter who puts on a good show. Such boxers are esteemed by promoters, television commentators, the general public and the boxing fraternity itself. All associated closely with boxing are familiar with boxers who were never the same, mentally or physically, after a hard fight with a superior fighter or a recognised champion. The oft-used phrase "they never come back" accurately describes the effects of the brain damage such fighters have sustained.

Long-term damage

The brain has a limited ability to repair itself. In particular, once nerve fibres are divided anatomically no recovery of function is possible. Stretched neuronal networks may recover but probably take several months to do so. Fortunately, the human brain possesses a considerable reserve of function in most areas of brain activity. This reserve will differ from individual to individual and from function to

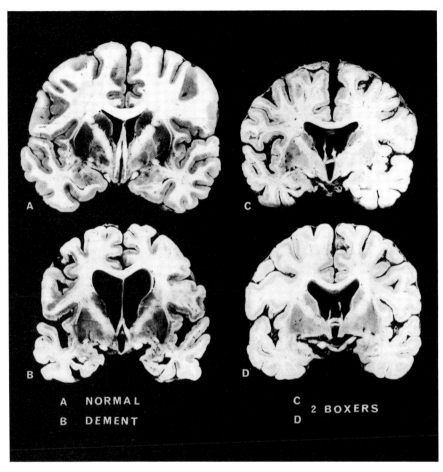

Figure 7
Coronal slice from 4 brains labelled A, B, C, D.

A is from a normal adult male,
B is from a demented patient with Alzheimer's disease,
C & D are from two 'punch drunk' boxers (suffering from dementia pugilistica).
The boxers' brains are smaller than normal with loss of the surface grey matter and inner white matter.
The fluid filled central cavities are larger than normal, but smaller than those in patient B who had Alzheimer's disease. The central septum in the boxers' brains are widely separated and torn. This is in marked contrast to the normal septum in A and the narrow stretched septum in B.

function. The effects of brain injury following a boxing match in which forceful blows to the head are sustained may therefore pass unnoticed and some boxers never show clinical signs of brain damage. The effects are, however, cumulative, so that the more punches that a fighter receives in his career the more likely he is to show clinical evidence of brain damage. Such signs are likely to appear towards the end of a boxer's career or they may appear some time after he has retired. This reserve of function that the brain possesses is affected by other factors. Age with consequent loss of neuronal function will reduce such reserve. The effects of advancing age may therefore become more obvious in the former pugilist. Other factors such as cerebro-vascular disease, hypertension, alcoholism, drug abuse and systemic neurological disorders may similarly expose deficiencies long after a boxer's career has ended. The former boxer, because of an already depleted reserve occurring when young, at the height of his cerebral prowess, may therefore suffer much more severely than a similar non-boxer from the natural ageing of the brain or from diseases of the brain.

When the neuropathologist is able to examine the brain of an ex-boxer and compare it with the brain of an individual of similar age and background, the cumulative effects of all the processes described may be seen. Typically, neuro-radiological imaging by computed tomography and magnetic resonance imaging will show the same characteristic pattern of visible change due to chronic repetitive brain injury. The boxer's brain looks smaller in bulk; the cortex (the surface grey matter) will be thinner, particularly in the frontal and temporal lobes and the fluid containing cavities (the ventricles) in the centre of the brain are enlarged due to disappearance of the surrounding white matter (see Figure 7). This is particularly well seen in the corpus callosum, a structure co-ordinating the activities of both sides of the brain.

Closer examination typically demonstrates that the damage is concentrated deep in the centre of the brain. The septum is seen to be torn and may be represented by a few shrunken tags of its former structure (see Figure 8). The fornix, thalamus and hypothalamus, structures that control basic functions of the body such as sexual activity, may be seen to be scarred and shrunken. The surface of the cerebellum, particularly the area around the foramen magnum and the posterior inferior surface of the cerebellum is atrophic and scarred with loss of the Purkinje cells vital in the control of movement.[7] On sectioning the midbrain the substantia nigra is a shadow of its former self with loss of pigment and neurons similar to that seen in Parkinson's disease (see Figure 9). Finally when the brain is examined under the microscope, diffuse scarring of the cortex, particularly in the medial temporal lobe, bears testament to repeated injury. Gliosis, the scarring that the brain develops, can be seen in the deep periventricular structures. Excessive deposits of iron on the surface of

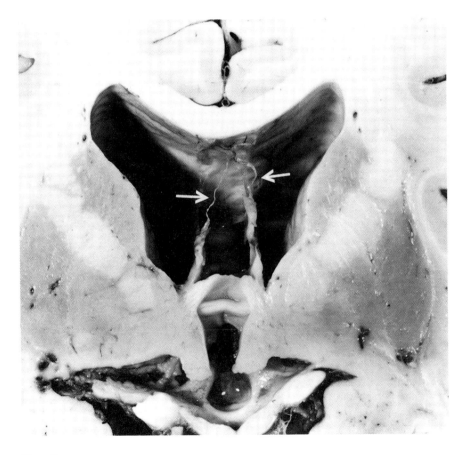

Figure 8
High power view of the septum in boxer's brain, Figure 7C (above). The two leaves of the septum (arrowed) are widely separated and torn.

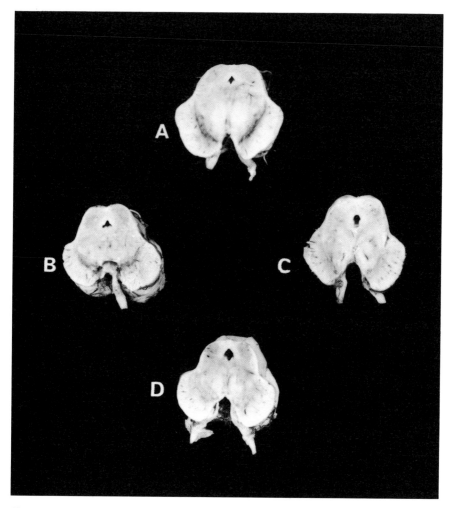

Figure 9
Transverse cut through the mid brain of an elderly non-boxer (A) to compare with B, C & D.
The normal darkly pigmented area (substantia nigra) is clearly visible in A. However, B, C & D show marked loss of pigment. The appearances in C & D are typical of those seen in severe cases of Parkinson's disease.

Figures 7,8 and 9 with kind permission of
Dr C J Bruton, Medical Research Council, Runwell Hospital, Wickford, Essex.

the brain and deep in the hemispheres is indicative of multiple bruises and haemorrhage that may have occurred in the brain recently or in years previously.

Of considerable interest in the pathogenesis of dementia, is the almost universal finding of widespread regional neurofibrillary tangles within the cortex. These are also found in the brain of elderly people or in those suffering from presenile dementia of the Alzheimer variety. Senile plaques which are seen with ordinary silver staining techniques in Alzheimer's disease are not seen in boxers' brains but recent work has demonstrated the presence of other plaques of beta-amyloid protein to be present.[8,9,10] Some boxers have died with Alzheimer's disease and there is growing evidence that repeated head injury is a risk factor in the development of that disease. The first neurological report on the delayed effects of boxing[11] concerned the case of a German amateur middle weight champion who 10 years after retirement, at the age of 28, developed Parkinsonism and dementia. The histological findings were those of Alzheimer's disease with amyloid vascular change. Also, the American boxer Sugar Ray Robinson had Alzheimer's disease listed on his death certificate although the primary cause of death was cardiovascular disease.[12]

The concentration of gliosis and atrophy in the medial structures of the temporal lobe are of special interest to the clinical psychologist. These structures, the hippocampus, amygdaloid nucleus, parahippocampal gyrus and fusiform gyri form a large part of the limbic system concerned with the function of memory and behaviour. It is not surprising, therefore, that the earliest signs of brain damage clinically are to be found in sophisticated neuropsychometric testing of memory and assessment of small changes in behavioural patterns that pass unnoticed by the boxer himself.

Can boxers be protected from injury?

Attempts have been made to protect boxers from brain damage by various measures. At best these can only be partially successful. The use of head guards undoubtedly protects against superficial injury to the face, eyebrows and ears but cannot eliminate the dangerous accelerating and decelerating forces applied to the head. Gloves are designed to protect the fists of the wearer and do nothing to prevent brain injury unless they are so large as to be unwieldy. Indeed, the bare fist prize fighters of the past were able to sustain very long matches because the force of the punches was less than in modern times. Padded flooring in the ring and padding of posts has eliminated the dangerous violent contact of the head with these structures. Early stopping of fights when one boxer is clearly out-classed or showing signs of neurological damage reduces, but does not eliminate, brain damage.

A proportion of the functional brain damage resulting from blows received in a boxing bout is recoverable. Prolonged periods of rest between fights therefore enable the brain to recover this proportion of the brain damage sustained before the next boxing bout occurs. Because of frontal lobe damage boxers tend to lose insight into their capabilities and their physical condition and are therefore not the best judges of the wisdom of embarking on the "come-back trail". The history of boxing is littered with examples of the price to be paid in damage to physical health by those who return to a boxing career.

In the case of boxers seriously injured in the ring, the greatest danger is that of death or very serious neurological deficit resulting from compression of the brain by an acute subdural haematoma. Immediate recognition of this complication followed by skilled control of the airway and rapid transfer to a neurosurgical centre where the clot can be removed and the coincidental brain swelling treated is vital, if more lives are to be saved. However, the mortality and morbidity remain high, despite skilled and prompt treatment.[2,5]

Boxing officials, in assessing a boxer's fitness to fight, place great faith in simple clinical examination and the use of monitoring techniques such as electroencephalography and the computed tomography of the brain. These methods are relatively crude and, will only detect chronic brain damage when already well advanced and in certain cases, irreversible. Careful and highly skilled neuropsychological testing[13] seems the only way of detecting brain damage in its early stages, although magnetic resonance imaging and radioisotope imaging may indicate acute brain damage soon after it has occurred. Chapter Three looks at the techniques available for detecting damage to the brain in more detail.

Injury to the eye

Structure of the eye

The eye is often likened to a camera, as it was indeed in the previous report of the Board of Science and Education working party on boxing (February 1984).[14] Useful although this analogy may be, it is not strictly accurate. The eye itself is a highly complex organ (see Figure 10). The more or less spherical tough outer coat, sclera, or white of the eye, is made up of interwoven collagen fibres. The cornea, a disc of clear tissue measuring about 12 mm in diameter, fits into the front of the sclera rather like a watch glass. The cornea is made up of very regularly arranged collagen fibrils, in multiple layers, set at exact angles to each other, such that the wave-length of light can pass through almost unimpeded. The cornea covers the anterior chamber of the eye, the iris, and its more or less central and circular pupil. Behind these structures

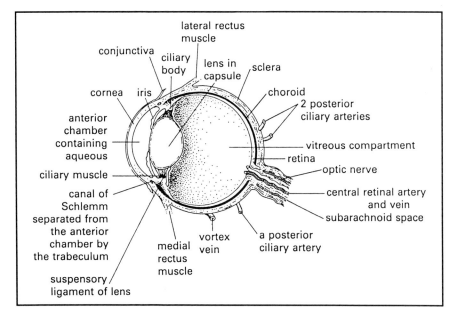

Figure 10
Structure of the eye in horizontal section.

lies the lens of the eye. Although the function of the iris is similar to that of the iris diaphragm in a camera, to enable differing amounts of light to enter the eye, the lens itself focuses in an entirely different way, by actually changing in shape and thickness, rather than being moved to and fro, as it is in a camera.

The sclera, or white of the eye, is lined by the choroid, which provides nutrition for the retina. Within the choroid lies the pigment epithelium and within the innermost layer of all, the retina. The retina contains approximately 130 million sensory units; 5 million cones, largely confined to the macular area or focal point of the eye and 125 million rods. Visual information from these sensory elements is channelled into 1 million nerve fibres in each optic nerve, high definition vision being present in a tiny central area of the visual field and increasingly ill-defined vision spreading out to the periphery. The cones provide high definition and colour vision and only work properly in good light conditions. The rods provide peripheral vision, giving information about movement and shape and work well in low light conditions.

The posterior chamber of the eye is filled with the vitreous, a unique tissue which consists almost entirely of intercellular glue with a little additional supportive structure. The anterior chamber of the eye is full of aqueous, a fluid manufactured from blood by an active process within the ciliary body. Although manufactured from blood under normal circumstances aqueous contains no red or white cells and is almost entirely devoid of protein. The rate of production of aqueous is normally accurately matched with the rate at which it can drain from the eye and the balance is generally such that pressure within the eye is maintained at between 10 and 22 mmHg, a level sufficiently above atmospheric pressure to prevent deformation of the eye by normal external pressure and yet not such that the blood supply to the optic nerve and retina is impeded. If the fluid pressure within the eye gets too high, satisfactory nutrition of the optic disc cannot be maintained and the patient develops glaucoma with death of nerve fibres and increasing visual loss, involving initially the more peripheral parts of the visual field.

The eye is contained largely within the orbit or eye socket. Although the walls of the orbit are made of bone, which is very thin indeed, the outer rim of the orbit is of very hard and strong bone and this, as well as the shape of the brow, nose and cheek, help to protect the eye from serious physical damage, particularly blows from above, under most normal circumstances. From below, however, the globe is significantly exposed and vulnerable to blows. If the eye receives a direct blow, it is in danger of sustaining damage which, depending on the direction and force involved, may range from the trivial to the extremely severe.

Mechanisms of injury

Three mechanisms are described by which a blow may lead to damage to the structure of the eye and its surrounding tissues. The first two are related to the punch itself and to the shock waves set up by the punch within the structures of the eye, a concept introduced by Courville[15] to explain the mechanism of brain damage caused by blunt trauma to the head. This concept is felt to be more than acceptable by ophthalmologists[16,17] since not only does the retina originate as an outgrowth from the brain but as in the brain itself the fluid contents of the eye are only too readily able to transmit shock waves. Thus a blow to the eye can cause damage to the cornea, iris and lens. Shock waves passing through the aqueous and vitreous can cause further injury to the retina, pigment epithelium and choroid, opposite to where the force was applied, resulting in retinal haemorrhages, choroidal ruptures and so on depending on the force of the blow.

The third mechanism in which damage is caused to the eye is that of equatorial expansion.[18] The compression of a fluid filled elastic-walled sphere from front to back will inevitably cause sideways (equatorial) expansion, to maintain the fixed volume of the globe (see Figure 11a). The vitreous is particularly strongly adherent to the retina in the region of the equator of the globe and to the ora serrata where the retina terminates. It has been shown by experiments with excised animal eyes that severe pulling forces transmitted to the vitreous base (the anterior part of the vitreous) can lead to the development of tears in the retina at the ora serrata. Such tears are accepted as being a typical sign

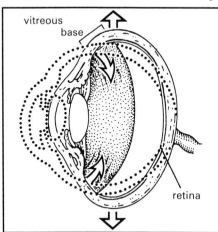

Figure 11a
Compression of the eye from a blow causes sideways expansion and traction at the vitreous base.

of blunt trauma. In some cases tears may extend over 90 degrees of the circumference of the eye and such so called "giant tears" are frequently reported in boxers. It has also been proposed that a blow to the eye can more directly push back the vitreous base leading to shearing and retinal tears developing as a result (see Figure 11b).

Some boxers and their advisers suggest that retinal damage only occurs if the eye is accidentally "thumbed" and it has been claimed that thumbless gloves would cause less injuries. However, thumbless gloves seem unpopular since the boxer cannot obtain sufficient grip for his needs when wearing them. In addition, it is not difficult to believe that a boxing glove itself, thumbed or thumbless, must by its relatively elastic nature, be able to transmit much of the force of a blow to the eye since the area of the glove, not impeded by the orbital rim, will continue to move forwards violently compressing the globe within the eye socket, somewhat like a piston in a cylinder. The globe in any case is unprotected by the orbital rim from beneath where it is particularly vulnerable to blows.

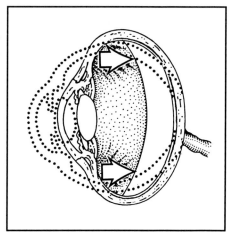

Figure 11b
It has been proposed that a blow to the eye can more directly push back the vitreous base leading to shearing and the development of retinal tears.

Conclusions

The brain and the eye are delicate and vital organs with a limited ability to repair damage received. Deformation of the eye due to blows sustained in boxing frequently leads to retinal tears and sight-threatening damage to other structures of the eye, including the drainage angle and the lens. Retinal detachments more or less inevitably develop following retinal tears if these are not accurately diagnosed and subjected to expert treatment. In young, non-myopic patients, however, there may be a considerable delay between a retinal tear occurring and the onset of retinal detachment. Retinal damage associated with boxing injuries is frequently so severe that treatment taxes the skills of even the most experienced of retinal surgeons. Very major surgical procedures may be required to save sight and a satisfactory outcome cannot be guaranteed. Cataract may also not develop for some time after concussive injury to the lens of the eye.

The force upon the brain due to the blows received in a boxing bout leads to movement of the brain within the skull and it is this movement that leads to damage to nerves, blood vessels and tissue. After an initial heavy punch that results in cerebral damage the brain is increasingly susceptible to further damage. Fortunately the brain has a certain amount of reserve capacity so that damage to its delicate structures may go unnoticed for some time. However, any process that further reduces the reserve capacity of the brain, ageing for example, may lead to the damage received through boxing becoming apparent. Little can be done to protect the brain from the damage received in a boxing bout and there is only a minimal amount that can be achieved through rapid treatment of injury. Boxing may therefore result in damage to the brain. Such damage may be cumulative and, unfortunately, once it has occurred there is no means by which lost capacity can be regained.

References

1   Atha J, Yeadon MR, Sandover J, Parsons KC. The damaging punch. *BMJ* 1985; **291**:1756-7.

2   Unterharnscheidt FJ. Injuries due to boxing and other sports. In: Vinken PJ, Bruyn GW ed. *Handbook of Clinical Neurology*. Amsterdam: Amsterdam North Holland Publishing Company, 1975;**23**:527-593.

3   Guterman A, Smith RW. Neurological sequelae of boxing. *Sports Medicine* 1987;**4**:194-210.

4   Strich SJ. Shearing of nerve fibres as a cause of brain damage due to head injury. *Lancet* 1961:**2**:443-448.

5   Cruikshank JK, Higgins CS, Gray JR. Two cases of intracranial haemorrhage in young amateur boxers. *Lancet* 1980:**I**:626-627.

6   Adams CWM, Bruton CJ. The cerebral vasculature in dementia pugilistica. *J Neurol Neurosurg Psych* 1989:**52**:600-604.

7   Corsellis JAN. Boxing and the Brain. *BMJ* 1989:**298**:105-9.

8   Roberts GW, Allsop D, Bruton CJ. The Occult Aftermath of Boxing *J Neurol Neurosurg Psych* 1990:**53**;393-398.

9   Roberts G W. Immunocytochemistry of neurofibrillary tangles in dementia pugilistica and Alzheimer's disease: evidence for common genesis. *Lancet* 1988:**ii**;1456-1457.

10 Tokuda et al. Re-examination of ex-boxers' brains using immunohistochemistry with antibodies to amyloid beta-protein and tau protein. *Acta Neuropathol* 1991: **82**:280-285.

11 Brandenburg W, Hallervorden J. Dementia pugilistica mit anatomischem befund. *Virchows Archiv fur Pathologische Anatomie und Physiologie und fur Klinishche Medizin.* 1954:**325**;680-709.

12 Merz B. Is boxing a risk factor for Alzheimer's? *JAMA* 1989:**261**(18);2597-2598.

13 Heilbronner RL, Henry GK, Carson Brewer M. Neuropsychologic test performance in amateur boxers. *Am J Sports Med* 1991:**19(4)**;370-80.

14 British Medical Association. *Boxing: Report of the Board of Science and Education Working Party.* London: BMA, 1984.

15 Courville CB. Coup-contrecoup mechanisms of cranio-cerebral injuries. Some observations. *Arch Surg* 1942:**45**;19-43.

16 Wolter JR. Coup-contrecoup mechanism of ocular injuries. *Am J Ophthalmol* 1963:**56**;785-96.

17 Benson WE, Shakin J, Sarin LK. Blunt trauma. In: Duane TD ed. *Clinical Ophthalmology.* Philadelphia: Harper Row Partnership Inc, 1985:**3**;1-13.

18 Maguire JI, Benson WE. Retinal injury and detachment in boxers. *JAMA* 1986: **255(18)**;2451-53.

CHAPTER THREE

Detection of
Neurological Injury

Direct observation of the intact functioning of living human brains is not possible and research workers and clinicians therefore rely on indirect methods of examination to detect damage resulting from head injury. The brain can be examined in terms of its structure, or in terms of its function and by imaging and non imaging techniques.

Brain function — non imaging

Clinical neurological examination

The neurological history and clinical neurological examination provide a somewhat unspecific mechanism, by which brain damage may be detected. Although elements of both are part of any general physical examination, special training and experience are required to detect the early, subtle changes involved in chronic brain damage. The neurological examination is generally directed towards testing a hypothesis generated from detailed history taking. Therefore a physician trained in neurological diagnosis who also has first hand knowledge of boxing and boxing injuries is the most appropriate person to perform such tests on boxers. It is difficult to provide a definitive description of what constitutes clinical neurological examination as methods may differ between clinicians. However, the examination would normally include assessment of the boxers' mental state, cranial nerves, motor system, reflexes and sensation. Assessment of the mental state will usually take the form of both observation during the history taking and interview, and formal testing of memory, speech functions, visual spatial abilities, orientation, attention, and concentration.

Standard clinical neurological examination employed in the course of research into boxing injuries will differ somewhat from examination of boxers to evaluate their fitness to box which would include consideration of retinal detachments, for example. Evidence of brain damage on clinical neurological examination is indicative of quite an advanced degree of damage. However, a clinical neurological examination may well be normal when CT scanning or neuropsychometric testing shows undoubted evidence of damage. A 'normal' neurological examination does not therefore exclude the possibility of brain damage.

Neuropsychometric testing

Clinical neuropsychology is an applied science concerned with the behavioural expression of brain dysfunction. Its main role is to identify cognitive deficits which can be attributed to cerebral dysfunction, thereby contributing to the diagnosis of brain damaged patients. Neuropsychological assessment involves the intensive study of brain function by means of interviews and standardised scaled tests and questionnaires that provide relatively precise and sensitive indices of behaviour. Such standardisation and quantitative procedures enable the clinician to reach unambiguous conclusions. There is now wide agreement among neuroscientists that for certain conditions, neuropsychological investigations are more sensitive in detecting cerebral impairment than clinical neurological examination or other investigative procedures. This is particularly true for early types of dementia and the effects of recent mild closed head injuries — the type of injury likely to be sustained through boxing. There has been a plethora of studies on head injured patients in recent times and it is well established that even minor accidents may result in significant temporary cognitive impairment. Indeed, such patients may show deficits which are not revealed by clinical neurological examination, which may be normal when neuropsychometric tests are abnormal. The precision and sensitivity of neuropsychological measurement techniques make them valuable tools for investigating small, sometimes quite subtle behavioural alterations and this technique is therefore of great interest to those attempting to identify early signs of neurological damage in boxers. However, neuropsychometric testing requires highly skilled and experienced personnel trained to identify and interpret the results of such tests.

Electroencephalography

Electroencephalography (EEG) is used as a measure of brain function through registering the electric current set up in the cerebral cortex by the action of the brain. Usually the EEG refers to brain activity recorded by electrodes placed on the scalp, which reflects the electrical activity of large neuronal aggregates. The central features in analysis of the resultant electroencephalogram concerns the wave forms, their distribution, and the context in which they occur. There is, however, considerable interobserver variability even among experts in EEG analysis and many patterns previously regarded as indicative of abnormalities are now regarded as clinically insignificant. There are a number of considerations to be taken into account when interpreting reported results of EEG abnormality. First, EEG findings are not specific for aetiology but may, in an appropriate clinical context, suggest or confirm a diagnosis. Second, although there is an approximate correlation between EEG and pathological abnormalities the neurophysiological basis for the different abnormalities in EEG remains imperfectly understood and unknown in many instances. Third, the EEG cannot compare with imaging techniques such as computed tomography (CT) or magnetic resonance imaging (MRI) for detection or localisation of lesions. Finally, it should be remembered that EEG abnormalities are not generated by the lesion itself, which is electrically silent, but by affected yet viable nerve tissue in the vicinity.

Brain function — imaging

Magnetic resonance imaging

Magnetic resonance machines of very high magnetic field allow spectroscopic analysis of tissue in addition to proton imaging. This technique is very much research orientated, but altered Phosphorus - 31 and Hydrogen - 1 metabolites are demonstrable in brain infarctions and other conditions; there are, however, no data with respect to boxers' brain injuries.

Positron emission computed tomography

Positron emission computed tomography (PET) is a technique in which the scanning apparatus detects and localises the destruction of positrons which are emitted during the decay of certain radionuclides. This technique can be applied to demonstrate and correlate cerebral blood flow (using labelled oxygen) and metabolism (using labelled glucose). Early reports of the use of the tracer Tc99m-labelled hexamethylpropylene amine oxime (HMPAO) in single photon emission computed tomography (SPECT) appeared in 1987. HMPAO is a lipophilic compound whose distribution in the brain is determined by regional blood flow at the time of injection and remains constant and measurable for some hours. Perfusion defects may therefore be demonstrated by this technique in the absence of MRI and CT abnormalities. The detection of abnormalities is currently based on asymmetry between the cerebral hemispheres; however, symmetrical perfusion deficits may cause difficulty with interpretation. In addition a preliminary report of cerebral perfusion in amateur boxers[1] noted a natural asymmetry between the two hemispheres in young controls, such that the non-dominant hemisphere receives slightly greater perfusion than the dominant hemisphere at rest. This finding was supported by PET studies. Despite these difficulties the technique appears to hold considerable promise in the assessment of functional abnormalities following closed head injures.

Brain structure — imaging

Computed tomography

The mainstay of structural brain imaging over the last 20 years has been x-ray computed tomography (CT), and since Hounsfield's prototype scanner was installed in Atkinson Morley's hospital, London in October 1971, successive generations of machines have been developed and a modern scanner can produce images of the

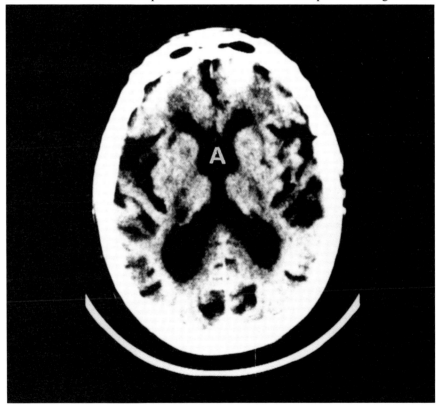

Figure 12
CT scan of the brain of an elderly ex-boxer suffering from dementia. There is severe atrophy of the cortex and white matter and marked dilation of the ventricles (A).

brain within seconds. The standard examination comprises a series of sections through the transverse axial plane of the cranium, using a slice thickness of 7 to 10 mm. The sensitivity of the system depends on the discrimination of different x-ray densities. The variation in x-ray density is simply a reflection of the distribution of electrons within tissue, since x-rays interact with tissue at atomic level. Modern CT can very clearly differentiate normal grey and white matter structures in brain substance as well as demonstrating detailed morphology of the ventricular system and subarachnoid spaces.

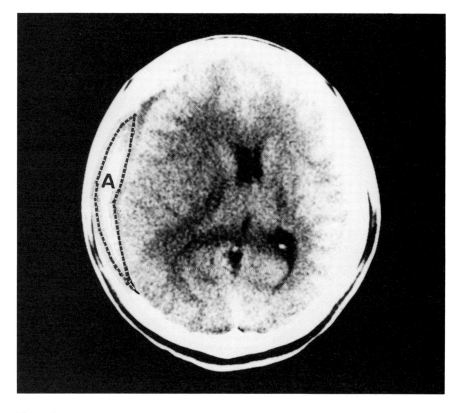

Figure 13
CT scan of boxer's brain: white stripe on the left of skull (marked A with dotted line) represents an acute subdural haematoma.

In chronic brain injury, atrophic processes are revealed by CT as localised or generalised areas of tissue loss with consequent enlargement of the adjacent ventricular system, subarachnoid spaces or both. The presence of a cerebrospinal fluid (CSF) collection between the leaflets of the septum pellucidum can also be detected, and may reflect septal tear. The endstage of most types of parenchymal brain damage, including traumatic, is represented by low density on CT scans, even if the acute injury was predominantly haemorrhagic.

In acute brain injury blood that has leaked from damaged vessels into the surrounding tissues increases in electron density during the process of clot retraction and serum extrusion and becomes bright on CT images. Thus it is clearly visualised, whether in the extracerebral spaces as a subdural or extradural haematoma, within brain substance, or in the ventricular system. Brain contusion results in local or diffuse swelling; the increased water content of the brain reduces the x-ray density of the affected tissue while areas of high density within such an abnormality indicate haemorrhagic contusion.

Magnetic resonance imaging

Magnetic Resonance Imaging (MRI) utilises the interaction of radio waves with mobile hydrogen nuclei (protons) in tissue water and lipids, while under the influence of a strong external magnetic field. Unlike x-ray CT, the appearance and sensitivity of the images are amenable to great manipulation by the operator. Such manipulation may alter the predominant features in the image from a simple proton density map to more complex images which reflect local nuclear interaction (T1 weighted) and those which depend on the effect of local magnetic influences (T2 weighted). For a number of reasons MRI is the modality of choice for most structural brain imaging, although not necessarily for acute brain injury where the speed, convenience, availability and accurate demonstration of haemorrhage by x-ray CT are advantageous. First, no ionising radiation is used in MRI imaging and the risks inherent in multiple x-ray CT examinations therefore do not arise. Secondly, although MRI and x-ray CT are generally equivalent in their ability to demonstrate morphology of the cerebral hemispheres, the ability of MRI to image in any plane is a particular advantage with respect to brainstem and cerebellar anatomy. Thirdly, although abnormalities of the ventricular system and subarachnoid spaces seen in

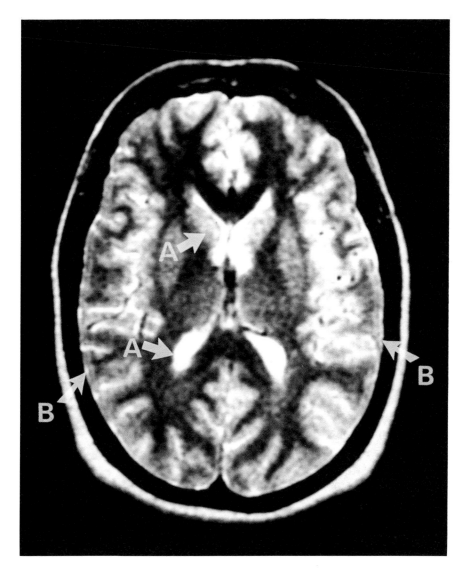

Figure 14
MRI of normal brain: note small ventricles (arrows A) and absent or narrow subarachnoid space (arrows B).

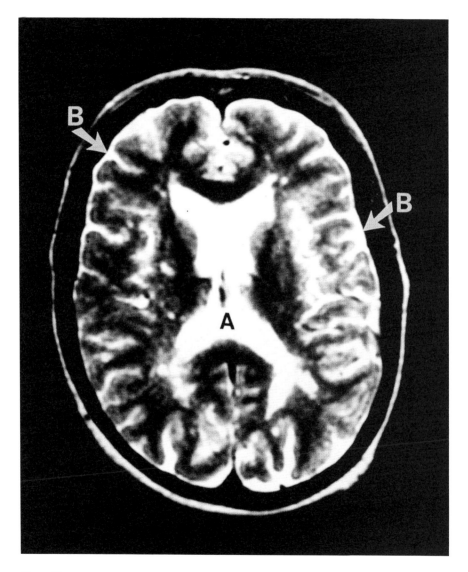

Figure 15
MRI following head injury: note large ventricles (A) and generous subarachnoid space (arrows B)
indicating atrophy of the cortex.

atrophy or hydrocephalus are demonstrated with both MRI and CT, MRI is more sensitive to parenchymal abnormality and may, for example, demonstrate lesions attributable to acute or old diffuse axonal injury when CT is normal. Fourthly, when haemorrhagic lesions resolve, haemosiderin deposits persist and are detectable by MRI but not by CT.

Summary

Imaging techniques such as computed tomography (CT) and magnetic resonance imaging (MRI) provide information on structural changes within the brain but are clearly not direct indicators of deficient brain function. Other imaging techniques such as positron emission tomography (PET) can be used to indicate functions of the brain such as blood flow or glucose metabolism. Non imaging techniques such as electroencephalography (EEG), neuropsychometric testing and clinical neurological examination also provide indicators of the functioning of the brain. Electroencephalography records the electrical activity of the brain and neuropsychometric testing measures the brain's behavioural product. All these techniques do have their limitations however, and do not enable anything but a crude understanding of the way the human brain works. In addition the relative costs and availability of the imaging techniques will have a bearing upon their use for detection of injuries in boxing; MRI and PET are of limited availability and more expensive than CT, for example. Research workers have therefore made it quite clear that for future progress in neurology, radically new techniques will be needed[2]. This chapter has outlined the various techniques available for detecting injury to the brain and provides the necessary background information to the research on boxers outlined in the following chapter.

References

1   Kemp PM et al. Cerebral perfusion in amateur boxers. Is there evidence of brain damage? Nineteenth annual meeting of the British Nuclear Medicine Society: Abstracts. *Nuclear Medicine Communications* 1991:**12(251-252)**;279.

2   Crick F, Jones E. Backwardness of human neuroanatomy. *Nature* 1993:**361**;109-110.

CHAPTER FOUR

Review of the Evidence

The 1984 report of the Board of Science and Education reviewed the available evidence for acute and chronic cerebral damage related to boxing. The report remains highly relevant to today's debate over the banning of boxing although much of the evidence presented in that report related to non UK boxers, and to those boxing before the introduction of strict medical controls. Further research into boxing has been carried out since the publication of the 1984 report, including a number of studies on UK boxers (see Table 4.1). A study carried out by Roberts in 1969[1] involving 300 boxers remains the largest study of damage to boxers and it is regrettable that such a large scale study has not been repeated using modern scanning techniques and neuropsychological testing.

The majority of studies carried out since 1984 have examined amateur boxers., with many authors attempting to illustrate the relative safety of amateur boxing. The issue of most importance to the BMA, however, is that of chronic damage to boxers, which may not become outwardly apparent until after the boxer's retirement. Unfortunately, none of the studies carried out has followed a cohort of boxers throughout their career which makes it difficult to assess what, if any, early predictors there may be for chronic damage.

Study	No.	Controls	Amateur/ Professional	Abnormal Neurological Examination	Abnormal CT	Abnormal EEG	Abnormal MRI
Brooks 1987[2]	29	+	Amateur	N/A	N/A	N/A	N/A
Jordan 1988[3]	9	-	Amateur	0	N/A	N/A	0
Heilbronner 1991[4]	23	-	Amateur	N/A	N/A	N/A	N/A
Haglund 1990[5a-d]	50	+	Amateur	1/47 (2.1%)	0/47	16/47 (34%)	2/47 (4.3%)
McLatchie 1987[6]	20	+	Amateur	7 (35%)	1 (5%)	8 (40%)	N/A
Sabharwal 1987[7]	4	-	Amateur	4/4 (100%)	4/4 (100%)	3/4 (75%)	N/A
Levin 1987[8]	13	+	2 amateur 11 professional	N/A	N/A	N/A	0/9
Jordan 1990[9]	21	-	4 amateur 17 professional	N/A	11 (52.4%)	N/A	9 (42.9%)
Casson 1984[10]	18	-	5 amateur 13 professional	5 (27.8%)	8 (44.5%)	7/13 (53.9%)	N/A
Drew 1986[11]	19	+	Professional	N/A	N/A	N/A	N/A
Kemp 1991[12]	20	+	Amateur	N/A	N/A	N/A	N/A

Table 4.1: Studies carried out since publication of the 1984 boxing report.
Studies are arranged in relation to the type of boxer examined; ranging from amateurs with little experience at the top of the table to professionals with much experience at the bottom of the table. The study by Kemp et al is an exception as it has used a scanning technique not employed in any of the other studies reviewed and can not therefore be directly compared to the other studies.

Abnormal Neuro-psychometry	Age range (yrs)	Career length (yrs)	Bouts fought	Comments
Boxers significantly worse than controls on 3/24 tests	15-27	1-13	2-96	Active boxers. Boxers measured against controls rather than standard norms for neuropsychometric tests. No correlations found between boxing variables (no of bouts, knock-outs etc) and impairment.
N/A	16-26	1-9	4-32	Active boxers who had been suspended for min 90 days due to a knock-out or excessive head blows.
Impairments in verbal and incidental memory post fight, enhanced executive and motor functions post fight	16-30	-	0-50+	Boxers tested pre and post match
Boxers had lower finger motor function than controls	26-43	1-17	0-180	Former amateurs. In all tests apart from EEG no significant difference found between boxers and controls. No correlation of any test bar neuropsychometry to boxing parameters. Finger tapping had significant correlation with length of career and number of bouts.
9/15 (60%) ≥ 2 tests, 3 had results suggestive of severe impairment	18-49	-	4-200	Active boxers. Abnormal clinical examination correlated significantly with increasing number of fights, abnormal EEG with decreasing age. Boxers significantly worse than unmatched controls in some neuropsychometric tests.
N/A	34-40	9-13	>100	Symptomatic boxers studied.
Trend towards deficient reading and verbal learning in boxers	<30	2-11	Amateur 14-184 Professional 0-10	Active boxers at early stage of professional career or still amateurs. Boxers measured against controls rather than standard norms for neuropsychometric tests.
N/A	21-66	-	-	Study carried out primarily to discover efficacy of CT vs MRI (all active boxers bar 1 professional).
12>50% tests 18>1 test	18-60	1-22	7-240	Mixture of former and active boxers. Abnormal neuropsychometry showed high correlation with abnormal findings on CT or EEG.
15 (78.9%) in impaired range on Reitan Impairment Index	18-25	-	Amateur 1-195 Professional 0-37	Active boxers. No of professional bouts/losses/draws showed high correlation with tests deficits. Controls and boxers measured against standard norms for neuropsychometric tests. 2/10 (20%) of controls scored in impaired range of Reitan Impairment Index.
N/A	-	-	-	Preliminary report with use of HMPAO SPECT, boxing group showed significantly greater abnormalities than controls although the researchers noted that this finding must be interpreted with caution until additional numbers have been studied. Further trial in progress.

Additional studies reviewed:

Jordan 1988[13],   Acute injuries only of professional boxers examined over a two year period in New York State.

Enzenauer 1989[14],   Boxing in the US army — incidents of hospitalisation recorded only.

Adams 1989 [15],   Histological study of brains of deceased boxers, 10 professional, 8 amateur and four who died as a result of boxing.

The research summarised in Table 4.1 is examined in more detail in this chapter. The findings of these studies are presented in relation to the methods used to enable comparison between studies.

Methodology

The various mechanisms for detecting brain injury in boxers which were reviewed in Chapter Three indicated that the techniques available differ both in what they can reveal and in their sensitivity. Neuropsychometric testing has frequently been employed in studies of boxers and would appear to provide a sensitive method for the detection of subtle injury to the brain. It is difficult to make direct comparisons between studies as there is no common battery of tests used by the various research workers. Studies have also differed in that some have compared boxers and controls with standardised norms for such tests,[4,10] whereas others have compared the results of boxers directly with that of controls matched for age, education, ethnicity and participation in sporting activities[2,5a-d,8]. The latter approach would seem most appropriate as it is possible that the former may be detecting differences in boxers from the general population rather than showing any particular effect of the activity of boxing on the brain. Certain research workers have used boxers in training who have not yet sparred or fought, and other individuals who show a desire to become boxers as controls[2]. Although such controls should remove any confounding effects of basic differences in neuropsychometry between individuals who take up boxing and other individuals it would be impossible to find such controls for studies of older boxers — matching for age in the detection of abnormalities in neurological functioning is a primary requirement. Other research workers have therefore opted for controls that are professional or amateur sportspeople, who are also subject to rigorous training and physical exertion[5a-d,8,11].

The studies range from those examining young, amateur boxers with limited careers to those examining retired professionals with a long boxing history. Current boxers as well as ex-boxers have been included in such studies. Most research workers have recorded a variety of boxing variables such as number of bouts or number of knock-outs to determine the effect, if any, on resultant brain damage. Haglund[5a-d], for example, classified the ex-amateurs studied as high matched or low matched depending on the number of bouts fought. This variability in the boxers studied makes direct comparison between studies somewhat difficult.

Brain function — non imaging

Clinical neurological examination

Many of the studies reviewed employed clinical neurological examination and evidence of damage to the brain has been clearly identified. Casson et al[10] found abnormalities in five of the eighteen boxers studied, three of whom had a clinical organic mental syndrome manifested by disorientation, confusion, and memory loss. Casson did note however, that in one of these individuals the abnormality found could not definitely be considered abnormal due to the age of the individual — 58 years. Haglund et al[5a] performed a routine neurological examination, alongside a "mini-mental state" examination designed to distinguish between dementia and depressive pseudo-dementia. Slight deviations were found in four subjects, one boxer and three matched controls. All subjects had normal "mini-mental state" test values. The authors concluded that these results suggested an absence of "punch drunks".

In the study by Sabharwal et al,[7] the four amateur boxers studied all showed abnormalities on neurological examination. Neurological examination showed memory impairment, slurred speech and forgetfulness in all subjects and the authors interpreted such results as clinical manifestations of dementia pugilistica. Jordan et al[3] studied nine boxers who had been suspended from competitive boxing for a minimum of 90 days due to a knock-out or excessive head blows. Of the boxers studied, three had experienced immediate neurological symptoms at the time of their last bout; at the time of study (1 week to 3.5 months after suspension) no abnormalities were found on neurological testing. McLatchie et al[6] in their study of 20 active amateur boxers found seven to have an abnormal clinical examination which correlated significantly with an increasing number of fights. The authors were surprised at the high number of abnormalities, and although they believed that the indicators uncovered by an experienced neurologist were valid, caution should be applied to some of the minor neurological signs as they were sought so intensely. The great majority of boxers with motor system disorders found in this study were quite asymptomatic and it would only be through longitudinal study that it would be possible to show that these signs were the forerunners of clinical disability.

Neuropsychometric testing

Neuropsychometric testing would appear to be the method of testing most widely used by those studying boxers over the past twenty years. This is in contrast to studies reviewed in the BMA's 1984 report where CT scanning predominated.

Brooks et al[2] carried out neuropsychological examinations on 29 amateur boxers and 19 controls matched for age, ethnicity and education. To increase the accuracy of matching, 11 of the controls were prospective amateur boxers (training without sparring), at the clubs from which the subjects were chosen. Tests were selected on the assumption that brain damage, if present, would be similar to that found in minor closed head injury. Therefore verbal and visuospatial memory, attention, information processing and motor function, and intellectual abilities were all assessed. Out of the 24 individual measures of performance, only three showed significant differences between boxers and controls. No significant effects were found when boxers' performance in tests was measured against a number of boxing variables ie intensity of exposure.

The authors discussed their results at length concluding that their research could in fact indicate that carefully controlled amateur boxing is indeed neuropsychologically safe. They noted that in those boxers studied, any individual receiving a severe blow to the head during sparring is immediately stopped from boxing and from sparring for 28 days. They believed this temporary cessation of boxing activity to be important in reducing neurological damage as in less carefully controlled situations boxers may spar frequently and unsupervised. In discussing the significance of their results, the authors considered that they may have used inappropriate tests or inappropriate or inaccurately matched controls. The tests were chosen on the assumption that any brain damage in amateur boxing would be of the sort found in minor concussion, representing deficits largely in information processing and memory. The authors also considered that the boxers studied only represented 39% of the group invited to participate. It is possible therefore that those who refused to take part had a subjective awareness of neurological impairment. In addition, those studied were largely successful in their careers (18/8 ratio of wins to losses); it is possible that boxers with a large number of losses may reveal greater damage.

In the study by Heilbronner et al[4] 23 amateur boxers were assessed immediately before and after an amateur boxing event. Of the 50 boxers assessed prefight only 23 presented for postfight evaluation; the authors stated that this was largely due to scheduling difficulties. However a preponderance of the boxers who did not present for post-fight evaluation had lost their bouts and were likely to be uninterested in remaining for testing. Compared with their prefight performance, boxers demonstrated significant deficits in verbal memory, but enhanced executive and motor functions. There were no observed differences between those losing or winning their bouts. The authors concluded that for a number of reasons, the observed abnormalities could not be directly related to boxing: the subjects examined were volunteers and as such may have been unrepresentative of boxers in general, and men who take up boxing could come from a population who already have such abnormalities. In addition, changes in autonomic arousal may impact memory performance and indeed motor speed and it may therefore have been the psychophysiological state induced by the fight that led to the observed differences. The authors noted that the four boxers with the most extensive fight histories demonstrated slower dominant hand tapping speed after a fight compared with prefight. It is possible that these boxers could have sustained enough head blows with subsequent brain dysfunction that their fine psychomotor speed was affected. These four boxers had remained amateur beyond the time when most fighters would turn professional and this may be why their deficits were more pronounced, similar to that often found in professional boxers. The authors concluded that to study effectively the neuropsychological impact of amateur boxing, further longitudinal studies would be needed that included rigorous examination of critical boxing variables, use of appropriately matched controls, and more appropriate tests.

In Murelius' study of 50 amateur boxers and 50 matched controls[5d], similar results to that of Heilbronner et al[4] were found, with the only significant difference being in finger tapping performance. None of the boxers were considered to have definite signs of intellectual impairment. High matched boxers (boxers who had participated in a large number of fights) were found to show inferior finger tapping in comparison with the other groups both with the dominant and the non-dominant hand. A significant correlation between inferior finger tapping performance, the length of boxing career, and the number of fights was found. The correlation with length of career was also significant in the soccer players used as controls: those with a long career showed a lower finger tapping speed. The authors postulated that this reduced finger tapping performance could be due to peripheral nervous and/or motor functioning, rather than central damage. However the fact that soccer players with a long career also had lower finger tapping performance would tend to point towards a central cause — soccer players are unlikely to have sustained finger injuries but face the risk of brain injury due to heading the ball. There were however, no significant correlations between inferior finger tapping and the other brain damage sensitive neuropsychological tests, nor with the clinical neurological examination, EEG or with the CT and MRI studies performed on the same subjects.

McLatchie et al[6] in their study of active amateur boxers found abnormal neuropsychometry in nine of the fifteen subjects examined. In several of the neuropsychometric tests, the boxers were significantly worse than controls. As with other research workers, the assumption was made that boxing may cause damage of the kind found in minor head injury and a battery of tests were chosen to detect deficits in learning and memory, and various aspects of attentional performance. The nine boxers considered to have abnormal neuropsychometry all had poor performance on two or more of the clinical measures and in three cases results suggested severe impairment. The authors concluded that their study had shown that in a group of apparently healthy, active young men there was neuropsychological evidence of abnormal brain function.

Levin et al[8] studied thirteen young boxers at the outset of their professional career. A control group of 13 athletes was matched to the boxers, although there was an observed difference in oral reading skills — boxers being less capable than controls. There was also a difference in the daily regimen of total physical activity undertaken by the boxers and the other athletes, with the boxers undertaking extensive training and activity. Ten of the boxers were re-tested after six months to identify any progressive deterioration. The test data related a trend toward deficient reading and verbal learning in the boxers. Although the boxers more closely approximated the verbal learning scores of the control individuals at the six month follow-up examination, their reading scores still tended to be lower. The authors concluded that it was conceivable that a subtle impairment in processing verbal material resulted from boxing in these young men. Other plausible interpretations included an association between self-selection for boxing and a subtle learning disability or at least subjective difficulty in reading. Even though boxers and control subjects tended to improve their performance or remain stable on follow-up examination, the authors noted that longitudinal investigation over an extended period might disclose signs of delayed neurological disorder. In contrast to other studies, the authors were unable to confirm an inverse relationship between the number of bouts and the level of performance on neuropsychological tests. However, they suggested that confounding of educational status and parental socioeconomic level with boxing experience, and the relatively few professional bouts fought may account for these negative findings. Although the sample size of the study was small the authors believed their findings raised the possibility that young boxers may escape disabling brain injury provided that their exposure in the ring is limited both in frequency and total duration.

In contrast to these studies is the work of Casson et al[10] who found abnormalities in at least one of the tests carried out on all 18 boxers studied. Twelve boxers had abnormalities in more than 50% of the tests. Boxers were evaluated against standard norms and therefore no control group was used. Thirteen of the subjects were ex-boxers (2 amateurs and 11 professionals), 2 were active professionals and 3 were active amateurs. An impairment index was developed for the boxers from the percentage of abnormal neuropsychological test scores. Boxers with abnormal CT scans had a significantly higher mean impairment index than those with normal CT scans; this was also the case with those boxers with abnormal EEG records. Of all the known boxing variables, the impairment index correlated significantly only with the number of professional fights and with age. The authors concluded that their results indicated that the longer the professional career the greater the likelihood of brain damage — a cumulative effect of multiple subconcussive blows to the head being the likely aetiology. They believed that neuropsychological tests had proven to be sensitive detectors of brain damage. The subjects studied performed particularly poorly on tests which measured short-term memory and the authors believed this confirmed earlier findings that suggest impairment of recent memory as a central feature of the organic mental syndrome of boxers.

Drew et al[11] studied 19 young, active licensed professional boxers and found that they displayed a pattern of neuropsychological deficits consistent with the more severe punch drunk syndrome of years past. The boxers were compared with a control group of athletes who were matched for race, age, and level of education. The boxers showed significantly more deficits than controls on all but 3 of the 12 tests carried out. Fifteen of the 19 boxers scored in the impaired range on the Reitan impairment index as compared to 2 out of 10 of the controls. The authors believed their study showed that active boxers, fighting under improved safety regulations, and with no known history of neurological deficits, were still suffering from symptoms of the punch drunk syndrome of years past, but with less severity, including deficits in abilities needed for effective academic, vocational, and social functioning. The number of professional bouts and the number of professional "losses" and "draws", showed high correlations with boxers' test deficits. The authors concluded that their study indicates that brain damage in professional boxers is an ongoing process resulting from repeated head trauma and is cumulative in nature. The authors believed that their results confirmed the common sense notion that although the number of professional bouts may be a good predictor of cumulative impairment, the extent of brain damage is primarily a function of the amount of "punishment" received. On the basis of their research it would appear that number of professional losses plus draws is a good index of this punishment dimension.

Neuropsychometric testing, unlike CT or MRI, is able to measure functional damage to the brain. It appears to be a sensitive indicator of damage and is likely to reveal signs and symptoms of neurological deficit before structural changes are detectable by CT or MRI. Most of the studies reviewed have selected tests on the assumption that damage due to boxing would be similar to that found in minor concussion. To this end, most of the investigators have employed tests of information processing and memory. Verbal learning and verbal memory have been found to be deficient in boxers as has hand tapping speed, leading researchers to postulate that boxing may lead to deficits in short term memory and in motor function.

Electroencephalogram

Unlike scanning techniques such as CT that reveal structural damage to the brain, the electroencephalogram(EEG) reflects neuronal brain activity. There is considerable interobserver variability in interpretation of results (ie different people carrying out the test may get different results) and the subject's physiological state can be the primary reason for the abnormality; hyperventilation, for example, can cause significant changes. In all the studies reviewed that have employed EEG, high rates of abnormalities have been detected. Even in the study of Haglund et al[5c], which failed to detect abnormalities by other methods, 34% of the subjects had abnormal EEGs. This could either indicate that EEG is a sensitive means of detecting traumatic brain injury or be illustrative of the difficulties in interpretation of EEG. In Haglund's study, two experienced clinical neurophysiologists evaluated EEGs independently of each other. The EEGs were classified as slightly, moderately and severely abnormal. EEG abnormalities were found in 25% (24/97) of subjects and controls: 32% (7/22) of the high matched (high number of fights) boxers, 36% (9/25) of the low matched (low number of fights) boxers, 20% (5/25) of the soccer players and 12% (3/25) of the track and field athletes. Statistically significant differences were found between the boxers' group and the track and field group and between the low matched boxers and the track and field group. There were no correlations with age or boxing variables; for example, number of knock-outs. However, when one of the boxers was excluded due to the likelihood of past medical treatment causing abnormalities in his EEG, the statistical difference between the boxers group and the track and field group was no longer present. The reliability of such results were discussed in detail with the authors concluding that an EEG difference existed between boxers and controls and that they could not exclude the possibility that it might represent a sign of brain dysfunction in some of the amateur boxers. It was emphasised however that no severe abnormalities were found in this study.

McLatchie et al[6] found evidence of abnormal EEG recordings in 40% of the subjects studied. The EEGs were examined by one of the research workers and independently by a specialist in electroencephalography. Abnormal EEG correlated significantly with age; the younger the boxer, the more likely he was to have an abnormal EEG. There was no correlation between an abnormal EEG and the number of fights. In their discussion the authors referred to the fact that EEG is outside normal limits in 10-20% of the population, with less mature brains the EEG is more likely to be abnormal. They concluded that a single EEG is not therefore the best method for diagnosing brain damage but that a series of EEGs showing an abnormality emerging over time would be of significance.

Sabharwal et al[7] found abnormal EEG recordings in three of the four boxers studied. In all other tests carried out on the boxers, all four showed abnormalities, which was not surprising as they were classified as being symptomatic of dementia pugilistica. It is, however, surprising that one of the boxers who showed abnormalities in all other tests should not have EEG abnormalities. Casson et al[10] carried out an EEG in 13 of the 18 boxers studied. EEG recordings were interpreted by independent examination. Seven individuals were found to have abnormal records. Every boxer who had an abnormal EEG also had impairment on neuropsychological testing.

It would appear from these studies that EEG may prove a useful tool in detecting abnormalities in brain activity due to trauma. However, there are difficulties in interpreting the results of such tests particularly where the boxers are being compared with standard norms rather than with matched controls. It would also seem that carrying out a number of EEGs over a period of time to detect any emerging abnormalities would provide a more useful assessment by this method.

Brain function — imaging

Hexamethylpropylene amine oxime, single photon emission computed tomography

Hexamethylpropylene amine oxime (HMPAO) single photon emission computed tomography (SPECT), like EEG and neuropsychometric testing provides a method of detecting functional changes in the brain. With regard to boxing it has only been employed in one study of amateur naval boxers. Early results of this study were presented at the 1991 annual meeting of the British Nuclear Medicine Society[12]. Twenty amateur boxers and 41 matched controls underwent SPECT imaging. The interpretation of the scans was undertaken by two independent observers. The control group demonstrated greater abnormalities than had been noted in other series and also revealed a significant asymmetry in cortical uptake of HMPAO: the left (largely dominant) hemisphere showed reduced perfusion compared with the right hemisphere — a finding supported by PET scanning. The boxing group showed significantly greater abnormalities than the controls although the authors noted that this finding must be interpreted with caution until additional subjects have been studied. To this end the Armed Forces are planning a large scale trial involving the boxing associations of all three Services. This study will assess the boxers' cerebral perfusion patterns on a sequential basis in order to assess for alterations with time. The results of this important study should be available in 1994.

Brain structure — imaging

Computed tomography

Computed tomography (CT) has been used by a number of authors to indicate signs of structural damage to the brain. Haglund et al[5b] carried out CT scans on 47 individuals who had been amateur boxers. The scans were independently evaluated by four experienced neuroradiologists for width and shape of the ventricular system. The boxers scans were compared with those of control athletes. Changes within the temporal lobes of the brain and the most posterior region of the cerebrum were found in one of the boxers with the remaining subjects and controls showing no abnormalities. There were no significant differences between boxers and controls. A cavum septum pellucidum (CSP) was found in 4% of the boxers and in 8% of the controls. It was suggested that the abnormalities found in one boxer could be explained by long term use of immunosuppressive drugs and corticosteroids; it was therefore impossible to say that such changes were due to boxing. Although a cavum septum pellucidum has been claimed by some to represent a sign of repeated head trauma, the authors of this study concluded that its presence in the track and field athletes used as controls, indicated that a CSP is more likely a normal anatomical variation and not a sign of earlier head trauma. It is interesting to note that although many authors have excluded from their studies boxers with a history of heavy drinking or of solvent abuse because of an association with brain atrophy, in this study boxers who had been identified as having long exposure to organic solvents/or of having a heavy alcohol consumption did not show any abnormalities on CT scans.

Similar results were obtained by McLatchie et al[6] who found abnormal CT scans in only one of the 20 active amateurs studied. The authors were not surprised by this finding as CT scans only detect severe degrees of chronic damage; this, they believed explained the well recognised abnormalities seen in professional boxers examined by CT. They therefore concluded that a normal CT scan does not exclude significant brain damage and cannot be used alone for assessing it. In the study by Sabharwal et al[7] abnormalities in the form of generalised atrophy were found in all subjects studied.

Although the study by Jordan et al[9] was primarily carried out to assess the efficacy of CT scanning compared to MRI, 11 of the boxers studied were found to have abnormalities on CT scans. The abnormalities of 3 of these boxers were verified as artefacts (faults on the radiographs which are not true shadows of the structures being x-rayed) by subsequent MRI scanning.

The study by Casson et al[10] revealed eight abnormal scans in the 18 boxers studied, a CSP was noted in three of these eight. Six of the eight fighters with more than 20 professional fights had abnormal CT scans as opposed to two of the 10 boxers with less than 20 professional bouts. Four of the five highly ranked or champion professionals had abnormal scans. The authors believed that the results of their study lent further support to the direct relationship between length of boxing career and the presence of brain damage. However in contrast to Haglund et al[5b] the authors believed that a CSP in a boxer should not be dismissed as a normal variant but should be considered a sign of encephalopathy.

It would appear from the results of studies employing CT that abnormalities are more frequently present in those with a long boxing career, particularly a professional career. In less experienced boxers and in amateurs the frequency of CT detected abnormalities is much lower. As CT only reveals structural damage to the brain and is not a direct measure of functional capacity its correlation with the degree of functional damage to the brain is limited. In fact by the time any damage is identifiable by CT it is possible that the boxer may already be exhibiting observable signs and symptoms of neurological damage.

Magnetic resonance imaging

Magnetic resonance imaging (MRI) was carried out in a number of studies. The number of abnormalities detected was low apart from in the study by Jordan et al[9] where abnormalities were found in 42.9% of the boxers studied. However, this study was primarily carried out to assess the efficacy of MRI compared with CT. The authors concluded from their study that MRI would appear to be the neuroradiodiagnostic test of choice in the evaluation of chronic traumatic anatomical lesions of the central nervous system in boxing.

Haglund et al[5b] carried out MRI scans in 47 of the 50 boxers studied. The scans were evaluated by two neuroradiologists trained in MRI interpretation and were compared with the results of control athletes. The MRI scans were evaluated for anatomical alterations and damage to the brain parenchyma. Two boxers were found to have evidence of changes in the parenchyma. Three control athletes showed anatomical changes: one soccer player and two track and field athletes. MRI did not demonstrate any pathological changes that were not seen with CT. In discussion, the authors believed that the MRI findings in boxers could not be related to earlier trauma with any degree of certainty. None of the MRI findings correlated with boxing parameters, for example, length of career.

In an earlier study by Jordan et al[3], MRI scans were carried out on nine amateur boxers who participated in the New York City Golden Gloves competition. The MRI scans were carried out on all nine boxers within 3.5 months of their medical suspension from boxing due to knock-out or after suffering excessive head blows. The MRI scans were normal in all cases. The authors felt that their results reflected the limited size of the sample and the fact that detection of acute or chronic lesions of the CNS by MRI is time dependent. For example, absence of MRI abnormalities is typical of patients (non boxers) suffering from post traumatic concussive syndromes. The authors therefore suggest that because of the proven ability of MRI to detect subtle parenchymal and extra axial traumatic lesions not seen with CT scanning, its use in the evaluation of amateur boxers should be pursued, with studies being done within 1 month of trauma so that these lesions may be detected.

Levin et al[8] undertook a study of 13 boxers and 13 matched controls; nine of the boxers underwent MRI. The images of all nine boxers were interpreted as normal by two neuroradiologists. Due to the fact that the subjects in their study were young boxers at the outset of their professional career, and not withstanding the constraints of the small numbers studied, the authors concluded that it may be possible that young boxers escape disabling brain injury provided that their exposure in the ring is limited both in frequency and total duration.

As with CT scanning MRI only detects structural damage to the brain and can not directly predict the level of functional damage. The studies reviewed indicate that MRI has the ability to detect damage that may go undetected by CT scanning. The studies have shown that care must be taken over the timing of scans in order that certain types of damage are not missed. It would seem that MRI may be able to detect structural damage at an earlier stage than CT, and may be particularly useful for identifying asymptomatic cases.

Additional studies

Acute injuries

Jordan et al[13] studied acute injuries among professional boxers in New York State over a two year period. It was calculated that 1.2 injuries occurred per 10 rounds fought — 0.8 craniocerebral and 0.4 others. Only acute injuries occurring in the ring during a competitive bout were included. Chronic injuries, such as traumatic cataracts, retinal detachments and chronic traumatic encephalopathy were excluded. Injuries occurring during training and sparring or outside the ring ie, not boxing related were also excluded. The information used for the study was obtained from report forms filed by ring-side physicians and results were therefore very much dependent on the accurate completion of such forms. The authors were careful to emphasise that their data should not be used to draw inferences about the development of chronic boxing injuries such as chronic traumatic encephalopathy and should not be used to comment on chronic conditions. The authors believed the recorded injury rate to be relatively low; however, it should be noted that all the injuries sustained were intentional and a legitimate part of boxing, unlike similar injuries occurring in sporting activities which are primarily accidental.

Hospitalisation rates

Enzenauer et al[14] studied boxing related injuries in the US army from 1980 through to 1985. The authors reviewed hospitalisations for boxing related injuries in US Army Medical Treatment facilities world wide. There were in total 410 hospital admissions for boxing related injuries. The average length of hospitalisation was 5.1 days US Army-wide, with 8.9 days average length of disability. Head injuries accounted for 68% of all boxing related hospitalisations but for a sub-group of USA army cadets constituted 81% of all hospitalisations. The authors concluded that the morbidity associated with military boxing made the continued promotion of competitive boxing in the military a controversial question.

Histological evidence

Adams and Bruton[15] examined the brains of 22 ex-boxers histologically to determine the frequency of recent or old haemorrhage. Four of these boxers had become comatose within thirty minutes of a boxing bout and had not regained consciousness. seventeen of the 22 ex-boxers showed evidence of past cerebral, cerebellar or meningeal haemorrhage which had occurred sometime during the boxer's life, although the extent of past haemorrhage was less evident in the amateurs than in the ex-professional boxers. However, the authors concluded that even in the ex- professional boxers the degree of cerebral damage, as measured by the amount of free-lying haemosiderin, was relatively minor and almost certainly could not have accounted for the extensive neuropathology that characterises the "punch drunk" state.

Such studies are indicative of the risks and treatment costs associated with boxing. The study by Jordan et al[13] revealed the extent of acute injuries occurring in one state within the United States and the study of Enzenauer et al[14] revealed the not inconsiderable cost to the US army of boxing through hospitalisation and lost working days. Adams and Bruton[15] concluded that the damage found appeared to be additional to the cerebral pathology normally associated with dementia pugilistica which suggests that processes in addition to those related to haemorrhage were responsible.

Damage to the eye

Evidence of serious eye injuries associated with boxing has been well established in the medical literature for the last forty years.[16,17,18] A more recent survey by Giovinazzo et al[19] of 74 boxers examined over a two years period when applying for new or yearly renewal licences, found at least one ocular injury in 66% of the boxers examined, and sight threatening injuries with significant damage to the angle, lens, macula or peripheral retina occurring in 58% of their group. Nineteen percent of their boxer patients had drainage angle abnormalities that could lead to secondary glaucoma, 19% had cataracts, over 70% of which were posterior subcapsular in position and 24% were found to have retinal tears. Giovinazzo and colleagues suggested various possible measures to reduce ocular trauma in boxing and to enable more satisfactory scientific studies to be carried out. Other research workers found ocular injuries in 5% (22/401) of soldiers hospitalised for boxing related trauma.[20]

Maguire and Benson (1986)[21] reviewed cases of rhegmatogenous retinal detachment (retinal detachments associated with tears as oppose to holes) in patients between the ages of 20 and 30 years from 1 July 1983 to 30 June 1985. They found 127 cases, 70 of which had a history of ocular trauma. Nineteen (27%) of the 70 had a history of a blow to the eye by a fist. Of these 19, 6 were boxers. Thus, as the authors state, "in the twenty-four month period, 5% (6 out of 127) of rhegmatogenous retinal detachments in patients in the third decade of life were in boxers".

Retinal detachments in boxers might be even more frequent but for the age of the contestants. Because the vitreous is well formed in youth, retinal detachment does not necessarily immediately follow the development of a retinal tear. With increasing age, the vitreous gel degenerates and becomes more fluid, leading to the early development of retinal detachment associated with retinal breaks. As Giovinazzo et al[19] have shown, 49 (66%) of a group of 74 boxers that they examined had at least one ocular pathological change in either the anterior or posterior segment of the eye and 43 (58%) of their group suffered at least one vision threatening injury. Bilateral vision threatening injuries were present in 21 (28%) of the boxers.

Conclusions

Table 4.1 reveals quite clearly the small numbers of subjects involved in the studies carried out since publication of the 1984 boxing report. The numbers involved make it difficult to extrapolate findings to the entire boxing population and many authors have noted this in their conclusions. It is also unfortunate that none of the studies have followed boxers throughout their careers and into retirement as this would enable an analysis of any progressive deterioration in neurological functioning. Regardless of such limitations, if an overview is taken of the available evidence, general conclusions can be drawn regarding the risks involved in both professional and amateur boxing.

Professional boxers

The studies reviewed confirm the findings of previous research and of the BMA's 1984 report on boxing — that professional boxers suffer from the effects of cumulative damage to the brain which may result in symptoms of the punch drunk syndrome (dementia pugilistica). The punch drunk syndrome associated with boxing has been acknowledged since 1928; it results in slurred speech, poor balance and loss of coordination with memory loss leading to dementia and premature death. The syndrome can develop years after the boxer has stopped boxing. The only study which appeared to refute the development of chronic injury was by Levin et al[8]. This study was carried out on professional boxers at the outset of their career and it may well be the case that if such boxers had been followed over a longer time period, deterioration due to cumulative damage may have been revealed. The authors suggested that neurological damage could be mitigated by reducing the number of rounds in professional bouts; as such, they would appear to draw the same conclusions as other authors, namely, that the damage suffered in professional boxing is cumulative in nature.

Although the studies of professional boxers reviewed here were carried out in the United States, it is reasonable to extrapolate results of such studies to boxers registered within the UK, as professional boxing is carried out at an international level. However, there may be differences in controls such as suspension due to injury and to the amounts of sparring undertaken in different countries which could lead to differences in the risk to professional boxers. The BBBC responded to the 1984 report of the BMA by stating that the research presented in the report related to non UK boxers and to boxers fighting before the introduction of strict medical and safety controls. The research presented in this report provides neuropsychometric and CT scan evidence of chronic brain damage in today's professional boxers regardless of improved safety and medical controls. It is also of note that the brain material used in neuropathological studies comes almost exclusively from the UK. The neuropathology of dementia pugilistica has therefore been derived almost exclusively from UK and not USA boxers.

Amateur boxers

The evidence for damage resulting from amateur boxing is far less clear as a number of studies found no evidence of chronic neurological damage in amateur boxers when compared with matched controls. There are of course limitations with such studies particularly due to the relatively small sample populations and most authors have stated that their results could not be extrapolated to all amateur boxers with any degree of certainty. The selection of suitable controls and the possibility that boxers may represent an individual sub-set of the population with regard to neuropsychological functioning need consideration in the interpretation of results. There are further difficulties in the interpretation of the studies reported here as the rules and regulations of boxing and medical controls may differ considerably between countries.

Methods of detecting injury

There is wide agreement among neuroscientists that for certain conditions, neuropsychological investigations are more sensitive in detecting cerebral impairment than clinical neurological examination or other investigative procedures. In the studies reviewed in this chapter, neuropsychometry detected functional deficiencies where structural damage was apparent by other test mechanisms and in certain studies detected functional deficiencies where no structural damage was apparent. However, the fact that those mechanisms for detecting structural damage (CT and MRI) were usually abnormal in those showing impairments by neuropsychometric testing is evidence that CT and MRI are good predictors of functional impairment.

In a study carried out by Jordan et al[9] to assess the efficiency of MRI compared with CT there were no instances where abnormalities demonstrated on CT scanning were not detected by an MRI scan. However, some abnormalities on MRI scans were not detected on CT scans. With MRI the brain surface is directly visualised in a manner that is impossible with CT; in addition, there is better contrast between areas of damaged brain parenchyma and normal brain parenchyma because the pathological processes involved increase tissue water that is more easily detected on MRI scans. Haemorrhage has characteristic intensity patterns on MRI scan (at least after the first one to two days) that persist for several months while characteristic CT density changes are present for only the first one to two weeks. CT is therefore more effective in confirming acute (24 hrs) severe head trauma, as MRI may not be able to detect damage at this early stage.

Further work is needed to establish the most appropriate neuropsychometric tests for detecting the type of deficiencies likely to be found in boxing, as the assumption that these will be similar to those found in minor head injury may be unfounded. Matching for education and for age are important factors in neuropsychometry although care is needed to ensure that educational abilities are assessed on factors that precede the boxing career which may already have had effects on intellectual abilities.

Cumulative damage

Common sense would point to the likelihood that damage from boxing is cumulative in nature and this would appear to be confirmed by the research reviewed. The research included in table 4.1 has been arranged in approximate order of career progress of the boxers studied, ranging from Brooks et al[2,] who studied young amateur boxers with very little experience, to Drew et al[11] who studied purely professional boxers with large numbers of boxing bouts. It can be seen from this table that, as the boxer's career and experience progresses, the likelihood is that structural abnormalities will be detected by MRI and CT increases. However, these are only broad observations as the full range of tests was not carried out in all the studies surveyed. None of the studies reviewed has followed boxers over a substantial time period and this would seem the most appropriate way of determining whether damage is progressive. It is well known that neurological performance deteriorates with age but the question is whether or not this process is amplified by participation in boxing.

Many authors have indicated that they believe there is a 'safe' level of participation in boxing. In other words boxing may be undertaken at a certain level or for a certain period without risk of long term damage. This is impossible to assess from the currently available evidence which has not compared boxers with a limited exposure to boxing over substantial periods of time. Due to the large number of variables that may affect the levels of neurological damage sustained by boxers, it may be impossible to predict with any degree of certainty a threshold level up to which an individual may box, without any risk of long term damage, even with evidence provided by longitudinal studies.

From the currently available research it would appear that damage to the brain is determined by a complex relationship of boxing variables such as length of career, number of bouts, number of knock-outs, ratio of wins to losses and so forth. The wide variation in exposure to risk between boxers causes difficulties in interpreting results of studies where the number of subjects is small — the largest of the studies being carried out was on 50 amateur boxers[5a-d]. There are also difficulties in finding suitable controls and in examining volunteer boxers only, as self selection may affect results. Ideally studies should insist on randomisation of subjects to remove the effects of self selection.

Future research

There is obviously a need for good quality longitudinal studies of amateur boxers to assess if there is any progressive deterioration both during their careers and on retirement. Martland, in 1928[22], estimated that almost 50% of boxers would develop the punch drunk state (dementia pugilistica) if they stayed at the game long enough. Roberts[1], almost 25 years ago, found that 17% of 300 ex-professional boxers had abnormal neurology. It would therefore be of great interest to re-examine the risks of chronic injury in professional boxers in the 1990s and to undertake a thorough examination of the risks of chronic injury in amateurs. Such research could determine more accurately the processes involved in injuries resulting from boxing and the most appropriate ways of detecting such injury. Current research indicates that neuropsychometric testing and IIMPAO SPECT provide sensitive means of detecting the subtle deterioration that may be occurring in such boxers. Given that registered boxers are required to undergo frequent medical checks and screening it would seem appropriate for the Amateur Boxing Association and the British Boxing Board of Control to assist with such research into boxing injuries to both brain and eye by recording the results of screening centrally. Such a register of acute and chronic injury amongst registered boxers within the UK would provide a more complete picture of the current risks to boxers.

As many of the signs of chronic brain injury may relate to personality or mood changes it would be of interest to undertake a sociological examination of boxers and their families. Rates of suicide or alcoholism in boxers may be illustrative of the effects of chronic injury as may subtle personality changes only recognisable by the boxer's immediate family. Once more the BBBC or the ABA may be able to provide information that would allow analysis of these possible effects of boxing injury. The BMA has prepared a questionnaire on boxing injuries and this is contained as appendix five to this report. It is hoped that doctors with boxers under their care may submit completed questionnaires to the BMA in order that further information on boxing injuries may be collated.

Notwithstanding strict medical controls, and neurological monitoring, there can be no guarantee that boxers will not suffer chronic or indeed acute neurological or eye damage once they enter the boxing ring. The studies carried out over the past twenty years do not provide adequate evidence for there being no risk of cumulative damage attached to participation in amateur boxing and provide substantial evidence for a well defined risk of chronic and debilitating damage in professional boxing. In certain circumstances, such as with amateur boxing, action may need to be taken on the basis of inadequate or incomplete data. Due to the risk of cumulative neurological damage boxing therefore remains unacceptable on medical grounds.

References

1   Roberts AM. *Brain damage in boxers. A study of prevalence of traumatic encephalopathy among ex-professional boxers.* London: Pitman, 1969

2   Brooks N et al. A neuropsychological study of active amateur boxers. *J Neurol Neurosurg Psych* 1987;**50**:997-1000.

3   Jordan BD, Zimmerman RD. Magnetic Resonance imaging in amateur boxers. *Arch Neurol* 1988:**45**;1207-1208.

4   Heilbronner RL et al. Neuropsychologic test performance in amateur boxers. *Am J Sports Med* 1991:**19(4)**;376-380.

5a Haglund Y et al. Does Swedish amateur boxing lead to chronic brain damage? 1. A retrospective medical, neurological and personality trait study. *Acta Neurol Scand* 1990:**82**;245-252.

5b Haglund Y, Bergstrand G. Does Swedish amateur boxing lead to chronic brain damage? 2. A retrospective study with CT and MRI. *Acta Neurol Scand* 1990: **82**;297-302.

5c Haglund Y, Persson HE. Does Swedish amateur boxing lead to chronic brain damage? 3. A retrospective clinical neurophysiological study. *Acta Neurol Scand* 1990:**82**;353-360.

5d Murelius O, Haglund Y. Does Swedish amateur boxing led to chronic brain damage? 4. A retrospective neuropsychological study. *Acta Neurol Scand* 1991: **83**;9-13.

6   McLatchie et al. Clinical neurological examination, neuropsychology, electroencephalography and computed tomographic head scanning in active amateur boxers. *J Neurol Neurosurg Psych* 1987;**50**:96-99.

7   Sabharwal RK et al. Chronic traumatic encephalopathy in boxers. *J Assoc Phys India* 1987:**35(8)**;571-573.

8   Levin HS et al. Neurobehavioural functioning and magnetic resonance imaging findings in young boxers. *J Neurosurg* 1987:**67**;657-667.

9   Jordan BD, Zimmerman RD. Computed tomography and magnetic resonance imaging comparisons in boxing. *JAMA* 1990:**263(12)**;1670-1674.

10 Casson IR et al. Brain damage in modern boxers. *JAMA* 1984:**251(20)**;2663-2667.

11 Drew RH et al. Neuropsychological deficits in active licensed professional boxers. *J Clin Psych* 1986:**42(3)**;520-525.

12 Kemp PM et al. Cerebral perfusion in amateur boxers. Is there evidence of brain damage?. Nineteenth annual meeting of the British Nuclear Medicine Society: Abstracts. *Nuclear Medicine Communications* 1991:**12(251-252)**;279.

13 Jordan BD, Campbell EA. Acute Injuries among professional boxers in New York State: A two-year survey. *The Physician and Sportsmedicine* 1988:**16(1)**;87-91.

14 Enzenauer RW et al. Boxing-related injuries in the US army, 1980 through 1985. *JAMA* 1989:**261(10)**;1463-1466.

15 Adams CWM, Bruton CJ. The cerebral vasculature in dementia pugilistica. *J Neurol Neurosurg and Psych* 1989;**52**:600-604.

16 Doggart JH. Fisticuffs and visual organs. *Transactions of the Ophthalmological Society of the UK* 1951:**71**;53 9.

17 Doggart JH. The impact of boxing on the visual apparatus. *Arch Ophthalmol* 1955:**54**;161-9.

18 Hruby K. Klin Monatsbl Augenheilkd. 1979:**174**;314-316.

19 Giovinazzo VJ, Yannuzzi LA, Sorenson JA, Delrowe DJ, Cambell EA. The ocular complications of boxing. *Ophthalmology* 1987:**94(6)**;587-96.

20 Enzenauer RW, Mauldin WM. Boxing-related ocular injuries in the United States Army, 1980 to 1985. *South Med J* 1989:**82(5)**;547-9.

21 Maguire JI, Benson WE. Retinal injury and detachment in boxers. *JAMA* 1986:**255(18)**;2451-53.

22 Martland H S. Punch drunk. *JAMA* 1928:**9a**;1103-1107.

CHAPTER FIVE

The Boxing Debate

The British Medical Association has consistently campaigned for the abolition of both amateur and professional boxing since the publication of the 1984 report. In undertaking the campaign the BMA has gathered a great deal of information on boxing. The BMA has debated with those who support boxing through the media and through organised debates. This section of the report looks at the arguments put forward in support of boxing and at how the BMA and others supporting a ban on boxing have responded to such arguments.

Acute injuries and deaths

In 1986 Steve Watts, a UK professional boxer who had had over 25 fights collapsed after losing a fight, developed an acute subdural haematoma and, despite neurosurgical intervention died. Steve Watt's death focused attention on the BMA's campaign, particularly when the neuropathologist found considerable evidence of previous brain damage in a boxer who was regarded as a competent fighter.

In 1987, a UK amateur boxer, Joseph Sticklan died from a subdural haematoma after losing only his second fight. Subsequently, kick boxer, Keith Gorton, (kick boxing is potentially a more dangerous discipline than boxing) died in 1989.

Since publication of the 1984 boxing report, information available to the BMA reveals that eight boxers have died, and six have survived only after surgery for intra-cranial haemorrhage, although three of these individuals have evidence of long term brain damage. Since November 1988, three boxers, Gary Mason, Horace Notice and Frank Bruno, have suffered detached retinas and two have had to stop boxing.

The validity of the BMA campaign in favour of a ban on boxing has therefore been reinforced by tragedies in the boxing ring. Since 1945 361 deaths have occurred in the ring worldwide, most of them caused by a single or multiple concussive blows.[1] Appendix 1 to this report gives details of the amateur and professional boxers known to the BMA to have suffered acute brain or eye injury since publication of the 1984 report on boxing. This list is by no means exhaustive and does not include those individuals who may be suffering from chronic damage. However, this appendix is indicative of the types of injury still occurring in both amateur and professional boxing.

In addition to this clear cut evidence of acute brain damage occurring due to boxing, studies reviewed in Chapter Four indicate that functional deficits related to brain damage are still occurring. Such studies using modern techniques have not been used for a long enough period to demonstrate the emergence of fully developed dementia pugilistica, but it is probable that some boxers showing early signs of brain damage may progress to this. The lack of large scale studies of large numbers of unselected ex-boxers makes it impossible to estimate the frequency of such brain damage. Given that it is this risk of irreversible disease in those who survive a career in boxing that is of most concern to the medical profession, collaboration of the boxing authorities in carrying out such a large scale systematic study would therefore be welcome.

Is boxing more dangerous than other sporting activities?

That injuries are occurring in boxing is obvious — but does boxing pose a greater risk than any other sporting activity? The BMA does not dispute that injuries occur in other sporting activities and has held policy calling for a national register of sports injuries and fatalities since 1983. Such a register would provide vital information for the introduction of appropriate measures to minimise the possible harm from any type of sporting activity, professional or amateur.

Those who support boxing have presented two statistics to refute the BMA's case for a ban on boxing — the low death rate per year from acute injury for professional boxers compared with other sportspeople and comparative figures for risk of injury in other sporting activities. However, in attempting to identify the relative risks of boxing to sporting activities a number of factors need to be taken into account. First, the fact that comparisons are usually based on acute injuries, whereas in boxing there is the risk of sequelae of repeated minor brain damage — a factor that is relevant in few other sports. Second, the number of individuals involved in the activity. The number of boxers taking part in fights over any given year is difficult to determine but will be far lower than, say, the number of individuals taking part in rugby. Third, the level of exposure to risk. A professional boxer may only compete in a few fights a year with each fight lasting on average less than half an hour. Compare this to the exposure of rugby players to injury, with each player taking part in a far greater number of matches each lasting for an hour and twenty minutes. If the number of deaths and injuries are viewed in relation to the numbers taking part and to the level of exposure it can be seen that the boxer faces a far greater chance of death or debilitating injury each time they enter the ring than does the rugby player (or any other sportsperson for that matter) when they step onto the pitch.

Comparative figures for risk of injury frequently presented by those who support boxing are based upon morbidity figures from the Sports Council's report on comparative injury rates for various sporting activities. The figures used by the Sports Council have been calculated from the Office of Population Censuses and Surveys (OPCS) General Household Survey data. The data for participation rates in sporting activities and accident data have been combined by the Sports Council to provide injury rates for sporting activities. However, as boxing has so few participants, the data are not at all reliable (only 32 men were recorded as having boxed or wrestled). It is also untenable to say that a sporting activity has a low risk of injury just on the basis of whether people have accidents when they are taking part. In the case of boxing it is the long term risk of chronic brain injury that is of primary importance. It is also unlikely that an individual who boxed would consider being knocked out in the ring for example, an accident — this type of injury may therefore go unreported.

Regardless of such statistics, an overriding point is that damage to the brain in sporting activities is incidental; in boxing, such injury is deliberate. Indeed, the clearest deciding factor in boxing is the knock-out which necessarily results in significant neurological injury. The issue of gravest concern to the medical profession is the risk of serious impairment in those who survive a career in boxing. This is the post- traumatic encephalopathy of boxers which results in a progressive and at times selective failure of brain function and this health hazard is almost unique to boxing.

Can boxing be made safer?

Common sense points to the likelihood that damage from boxing is cumulative in nature and this is supported by the research available. With this thought in mind many research workers have suggested that there may be a safe level of participation in boxing, whereby an individual may participate for a given time period without risking chronic injury. However, it would appear that chronic damage to the brain results from a complex combination of variables such as length of career, number of bouts, number of knock-outs and ratio of wins to losses. The wide variation in exposure to risk between the boxers studied therefore makes it impossible to predict any safe level of participation. Even if further longitudinal studies were carried out, with boxing variables carefully recorded, it would still seem both unlikely, and in practice unfeasible, for chronic injury to be eliminated by limiting participation. The use of systematic testing to detect as soon as possible when chronic damage has occurred and to then recommend early retirement cannot undo the damage already sustained although it would reduce the risk of progression as a result of further damage. With regard to severe acute injury, this can occur early in the career of an amateur and it follows that no regulations can exclude the possibility of this type of brain damage.

Much has also been said about reducing injury in the ring by the use of head guards, heavier gloves and other such mechanisms. However, it is the changes in acceleration to the head as a whole that tears the blood vessels, not the impact with the glove. More importantly, the introduction of measures intended to reduce the force of blow to the head are of little practical value if the minimum force needed to sustain either chronic or acute brain damage is not known.

In 1983 the Journal of the American Medical Association[2] proposed measures to limit secondary brain damage that may occur due to an accumulating acute intracranial haematoma and subsequent brain swelling. These proposals were later detailed in an article by Corsellis[3] published in the British Medical Journal. Most recently such measures have been proposed by the British Boxing Board of Control in the light of the case of Michael Watson, the UK boxer who sustained acute brain damage during a WBO super-middleweight title in September 1991. Michael Watson suffered an acute subdural haemorrhage — bleeding from a torn blood vessel on the surface of the brain. The damage caused by this type of injury may take a while to develop explaining Michael Watson's ability to walk back to his corner and appear lucid for a short time after the bout. When he eventually became unconscious this was due to pressure inside the skull from the enlarging clot. The rising pressure reduced the blood and oxygen supply to the entire surface of the brain — hence the widespread, progressive damage which ensued. By ventilating the unconscious boxer, administering drugs to reduce brain swelling and by rapid transfer to a neurosurgical unit the delay before damaging pressure has produced irreversible secondary brain damage can be minimised. This kind of life support treatment is the province of anaesthetists, a speciality in which ring-side doctors often lack specialist training. It is possible therefore that if Michael Watson had had a fully equipped anaesthetist at the ring-side he would not have suffered such a great degree of damage to his brain. However, even the best centres for treatment of acute intracranial haematoma still have considerable mortality and many of the survivors remain disabled. In addition, such controls only deal with medical attention after injury has occurred and cannot prevent this initial damage occurring. There is no evidence to suggest that boxing is any safer today than it was when the BMA started its campaign.

Measures to improve safety in the ring have therefore been introduced but in spite of these brain damage, both acute and chronic, is still occurring. Given that there are risks of brain and eye damage attached to participation in boxing at all levels, boxers, and where relevant, their parents, should be made aware of such risks. Information on chronic and acute injury should be provided in printed form to all participants, either when they are licenced or at each medical examination before a fight, in order that they may assess the risks to which they are exposed.

Boxing and children

At the 1992 Annual Representatives Meeting of the BMA, a motion was passed stating, *that as the next stage of our campaign against boxing we should seek a ban on children below the age of consent from boxing.* The BMA is therefore particularly interested in boxing in those under the age of 16. Whilst young boxers do not have as powerful a punch as mature boxers, young boxers have been shown to exhibit early evidence of brain damage in some studies (see table 4.1). This danger was highlighted in 1987 by the death of a 15 year old amateur boxer, Joseph Sticklan, due to brain damage after his second fight. The BMA believes that children may not be capable of making rational decisions about the dangers of boxing and that encouraging their participation is irresponsible and unethical. Nevertheless, whilst

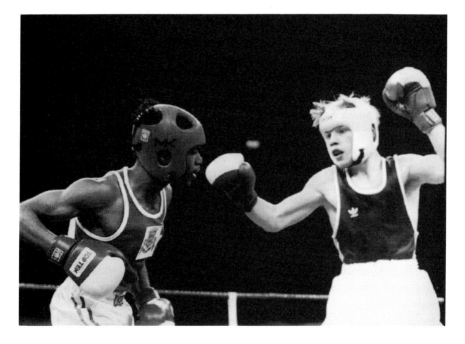

Figure 16
The use of head guards protects against superficial injury but cannot eliminate the dangerous accelerating and decelerating forces applied to the head.

boxing in those under the age of 16 remains legal, parents should be required to participate in consent and both the boxer and their parents should be informed fully of the risks. Information should be in writing, referring to both acute and chronic brain damage and acute eye injury.

Boxing by youths has been defended by some on the grounds that it disciplines boys who are underprivileged and provides a means of self-improvement. Today, however, there are many sports, such as athletics, swimming, judo and football that provide such discipline and, for some, a successful professional career. The BMA is aware that a number of local authorities have considered the position of boxing within their area particularly in relation to funding for boxing activities. Local authorities should be given support in providing alternative recreational facilities and should be encouraged to direct resources at forms of recreation that do not present risk of brain injury in children. In particular local authorities should consider whether the use of local authority or school facilities for boxing matches is appropriate. The Government, through the recently formed Department of National Heritage, should give consideration to how leisure facilities for the young may be improved, particularly in inner city areas.

It would appear that there has been a decline, for whatever reason, in boxing amongst children over the past ten years. The primary bodies involved in the organisation of boxing in young children are the Amateur Boxing Association (ABA), the Schools Amateur Boxing Association (SABA) and the National Association of Boys Clubs (NABC). Anecdotal evidence from the ABA suggests that the number of children now boxing has fallen dramatically in the last 10 years. Figures from the NABC reveal that of the 1920 clubs affiliated to them 260 are recognised amateur boxing clubs and that entries for the last NABC annual national boxing championships totalled only 166 boys under the age of 16. As far as the BMA is aware boxing does not form a regular part of physical education in the public or comprehensive school system within the UK. Although the NABC promote boxing within their affiliated clubs, a 1990 Her Majesty's Inspectorate report on the NABC designated boxing as *an inappropriate youth activity*.[4]

The organisation and control of boxing in the under 16s is somewhat unclear and in order to rectify this situation it has been proposed by the Sports Council[5] that a youth commission be set up under the auspices of the Amateur Boxing Association to co-ordinate the participation of children in boxing.

Boxing and the Armed Forces

There has been a long tradition of boxing in the Armed Forces both within the UK and within the United States. In a 1989 study of the American Army[6] the authors concluded that the morbidity associated with military boxing reported in their study made the continued promotion of competitive boxing in the military a controversial question. Since this time the question of boxing in the military has continued to be debated within American military journals. Within the UK a study of boxing injuries in the Army for the period 1969-1980 was published in 1983[7] and research continues on service boxers at the Department of Nuclear Medicine, Royal Naval Hospital, Haslar[8], where a large scale tri-service study has commenced to assess the cerebral perfusion patterns of amateur boxers. This study has the full support of the boxing associations of the Armed Forces which should provide sufficient numbers to be able to reach a conclusive outcome.

Although boxing is voluntary in the Armed Forces with no official restrictions on participation, anecdotal evidence suggests that it is discouraged among air crew in the Royal Air Force. There would therefore appear to be some acknowledgement that neurological damage may result from participation in boxing.

The role of boxing in the Armed Forces is obviously questionable. It would seem inappropriate to have boxing matches as part of military training when there is the risk of acute or chronic brain injury. It is also difficult to envisage what boxing can provide in military training that other forms of physical activity and training cannot; it would appear unlikely that the benefits of participation in boxing can outweigh the risks.

Boxing and the law

In February 1992 a Court of Appeal ruled that five homosexual sado-masochists were not entitled to consent to being assaulted.[9] The five men were convicted on assault and indecency charges. In commenting on this case, the general secretary of Liberty (the Civil rights campaigning body in the UK) said that the natural conclusion of such a judgment, from prosecutions under the 1861 Offenses Against the Person Act, was that other activities between consenting adults which led to injury would be illegal, including professional boxing. The House of Lords upheld the decision in

March 1993, several of their Lordships commented on the anomalous status of boxing. An analysis of the law in relation to boxing leads to the conclusion that a key consideration which the courts took into account in deciding whether boxing was lawful was the likelihood of injury. The law relating to boxing is based upon an assumption as to the lack of permanent harm. Therefore, if it can be demonstrated that the health of participants is endangered by the blows they receive, then the assumptions upon which the law's approach to boxing rests are substantially undermined.

In previous cases it has been stated that consent cannot render innocent what is dangerous and that there is a public interest in the health of the contestants. This would tend to indicate that if it can be established that there is in a boxing contest a significant danger of permanent injury arising, then the basis upon which boxing has been held not to be criminal but to be a lawful sport, "intended to give strength, skill and activity", falls away.

The ABA and BBBC are the two self regulating bodies which are responsible for organising boxing competitions in the UK. The extent of their potential liability to a registered boxer injured in one of their competitions is uncertain. However, one may say that, as a minimum, if a boxer were caused serious foreseeable injury due to the exacerbation of a pre-existing injury or condition, then if the regulatory body were aware or ought to have been aware of the existence of that pre-existing injury there would be potential liability in negligence. The type of injuries that may occur in boxing contests can lead to the need for long term and costly medical treatment. As the bodies responsible for the organisation of boxing contests, it would seem appropriate that the BBBC and the ABA make provision for such treatment costs, particularly where long term rehabilitation is required. The families of boxers suffering such injuries should also receive some form of support, financial or otherwise.

Consequences of making boxing illegal

Those supporting boxing claim that if boxing were made illegal there would be an increased incidence of injuries due to boxing continuing illegally, and without strict medical controls. However, anecdotal evidence indicates that in countries where boxing has been banned (Sweden, Iceland, Norway), this has not been the case. It would also seem an inappropriate assumption that laws should not be introduced because some individuals will break them.

The financial argument

The possibility of earning large sums of money for winning or losing a fight cannot be said to be inconsequential and is most worrying where there is a danger of financial considerations taking precedence over medical/safety considerations. Defenders of boxing frequently state that it offers working class boys the chance to 'better themselves' but all too frequently it is the promoters, sponsors and managers who make the money, often at the expense of the boxer's health. The argument is also put forward that boxers are fully aware of the risks that they take on entering the ring. This is not as categoric as it may seem; in particular the dangers of developing the long term brain damage known as dementia pugilistica (the punch drunk syndrome) are not well known and are frequently considered a danger of the past, visible in older boxers only because the current more stringent regulations were not in place when they began fighting.

At present, television provides the main source of revenue for boxing since most hall attendance fees do not cover the cost of an important match. It would seem appropriate for television coverage of boxing to carry information on the damage that is occurring during the contest. Commentators should be more honest in their description of the processes occurring. Phrases such as "out on their feet" for example, gloss over the fact that the individual concerned has suffered damage to the brain that has led to loss of control of motor functions. The sensationalism surrounding matches should cease because the mass media has a responsibility to both the boxers and the public to provide accurate reporting of such events.

However, the effects of increased awareness of the injuries relating to boxing and the continued efforts of the BMA and others, have been to alter views towards boxing as a 'sport'. It is recognised by certain individuals and companies that boxing no longer projects a positive image and in some countries there is now difficulty in finding sponsors for amateur and professional boxing. At the recent world championships in Australia, for example, several sponsors declined to support the event. Sponsors of boxing matches should therefore consider whether they wish their products to be associated with boxing. This is of particular relevance to charities and other bodies that raise funds through charity boxing matches, often involving young people.

International opposition to boxing

Even before the publication of the BMA's 1984 report, the Journal of the American Medical Association had published a powerful editorial calling for a ban on boxing in the light of the available medical evidence.[10] The editorial stated: *Boxing, as a throwback to uncivilised man, should not be sanctioned by any civilised society.* The Journal of the American Medical Association has since this time published a variety of papers and reports on boxing[2,6,11,12,13], including two more editorials calling for boxing to be banned.[14,15]

In 1987 the Secretary of the International Olympic Committee, Antonio Saramanche, stated his belief that boxing would be removed from the Olympic Games within the next 20 years. The BMA has offered to provide evidence to the Medical Committee of the Olympic Association on the risks associated with boxing on a number of occasions. The Medical Committee of the Olympic Association is currently considering the inclusion of boxing within the Olympic games and in 1992 took evidence from an individual UK medical expert regarding the injuries sustained through boxing. Once more the BMA offered its assistance with this enquiry.

At the 1991 ARM a meeting was held to agree a common approach to seeking a ban on boxing at the Commonwealth Games. At this meeting 12 medical associations (a full list is given in Appendix 2), including the Australian Medical Association and the Canadian Medical Association, signed the following joint statement:

"The undersigned National Medical Associations express the concerns of the medical profession regarding the dangers of boxing and believe that ultimately it should cease to exist. Modern medical technology demonstrates beyond doubt that chronic brain damage is caused by the recurrent blows to the head experienced by all boxers, amateur and professional alike. As long as it is legal to hit an opponent above the neck, there are no safety precautions which can be taken to prevent this damage."

The statement was endorsed by the Commonwealth Medical Association who, in line with the World Medical Association, oppose both amateur and professional boxing. Boxing has been banned in Sweden, Iceland and Norway and the BMA is aware of support for a ban on boxing within Europe, amongst the Irish, Danish, Finnish, Portuguese, German and Belgium medical associations.

Doctors' involvement in boxing

Doctors are involved in both the medical evaluation of boxers and in their treatment when injured. Before boxers may participate in a boxing match they need to be examined by a doctor who will certify them fit to box and it is this matter that has caused concern amongst some doctors. Guidance on carrying out such examinations was published in the American journal "Military Medicine".[16]

The Medical Ethics Committee of the BMA has discussed the requirement for Armed Forces doctors, who object to boxing matches, to carry out prefight examinations. The Medical Ethics Committee advised that doctors should make it clear that they can in no way predict the damage that may occur during the fight and that all that they can do is state that at the time of examination they found no evidence of a pre-existing condition which would absolutely preclude boxing. The BMA has further advised that a full explanation of the doctor's objections to boxing as a sport should be given to his commanding officer and that the matter should be handled through the recognised appeals procedure. Some doctors who feel strongly on the matter have considered resigning from the forces, rather than having anything to do with boxing matches. Although this is an extreme measure, it may be the only solution in cases where doctors consider that examination facilities or the way the sport is practised do not minimise the risk of severe injury.

Any doctor who is required to carry out pre-fight examinations of boxers should be provided with adequate time and facilities by which to carry these out effectively. Members of the profession should outline the risks inherent in boxing to the boxer and, if relevant, to their parents. However, any doctor's certification of a boxer as fit to box can provide no guarantee or indicator of the likelihood of acute or chronic injury occurring during the forthcoming fight. Conscientious objection should be sufficient reason for refusal to carry out such examinations although the doctor should refer the individual boxer to another physician.

Summary

The BMA's policy opposing both amateur and professional boxing has provided the basis for a high profile campaign to highlight the dangers associated with boxing. In pressing for an ultimate ban the BMA has gathered a great deal of information on all aspects of boxing. There has been much support for the BMA's work from the international medical community and from organisations, such as those representing young people, and individuals. This opposition is not based on moral considerations but upon medical evidence that reveals the risk not only of acute injury but also of chronic damage in those who survive a career in boxing. It is difficult for the BMA to obtain detailed information on all the injuries occurring among modern boxers. However, by monitoring reports in the media it has been possible to identify most recent fatal and serious injuries.(Appendix 1).

Over the ten years of the campaign there has been a notable change in media coverage of boxing. It is now commonplace for the media to report on the ongoing debate regarding the safety of boxing and the BMA's views have been reported by sports journalists and medical journalists alike. The case of Michael Watson brought about increased press interest in the arguments surrounding the safety of boxing and stimulated considerable concern. The BMA's campaign has therefore been successful in achieving this apparent change in attitude towards boxing and the damage that it may cause.

There are certain areas in which the BMA has taken a particular interest — boxing among young children and boxing in the Armed Forces — and these areas provide a particular focus for the BMA's campaign at present. A number of new areas of interest have been raised by the steering group's deliberations. The examination of the legality of boxing raises a particularly interesting question about the outcome of any legal case taken up by a boxer suffering dementia pugilistica (punch drunk syndrome) and there is perhaps further scope for examination of the doctor's role and legal responsibility in examining boxers both prior to and after boxing bouts. The BMA has therefore kept a watching brief on boxers and boxing in general, and maintains an interest in new research into boxing injuries.

This chapter has provided a brief overview of the BMA's work in attempting to achieve a ban on boxing and has highlighted issues of particular interest to the BMA. However, the main body of this report has focused upon research evidence for boxing related injuries. The BMA believes that there is now sufficient evidence for the risks of brain injury associated with boxing for the Secretary of State at the Department of National Heritage to call for an independent enquiry into these risks.

This British Medical Association study has found further evidence to support the conclusions of the 1984 Boxing Report. Acute and chronic injury to both brain and eye continue to occur in both amateur and professional boxers and, as such, the activity of boxing cannot be justified on health and safety grounds as an appropriate or legitimate 'sport'. The Association therefore recommends that the campaign to achieve a ban on both professional and amateur boxing should continue with renewed vigour.

References

1 Ryan A J. Intracranial Injuries Resulting from Boxing: A Review (1918-1985). *Clinics in Sports Medicine* 1987:**6(1)** supplemented by information contained in Appendix 1 of this report.

2 Council on Scientific Affairs. Brain Injury in boxing. *JAMA* 1983:**249(2)**;254-7.

3 Corsellis JAN. Boxing and the brain. *BMJ* 1989:**298**;105-9.

4 Department of Education and Science. *HM Inspectors Report on the National Association of Boys Clubs*. London: HMSO, 1990.

5 Sports Council. *Review of Amateur Boxing*. London: Sports Council, 1992.

6 Enzenauer RW, Montrey JS, Enzenauer RJ, Mauldin WM. Boxing related injuries in the US Army, 1980 through 1985. *JAMA* 1989:**261(10)**;1463-6.

7 Oelman BJ, Rose CME, Arlow KJ. Boxing injuries in the army. *JR Army Med Corps* 1983:**129**;32-37.

8 Kemp PM et al, Cerebral perfusion in amateur boxers. Is there evidence of brain damage? Nineteenth annual meeting of the British Nuclear Medicine Society: Abstracts. *Nuclear Medicine Communications* 1991:**12(251-252)**;279.

9 Convictions for sado-masochist upheld. Times 20 February 1992;6.

10 Lundberg GD. Boxing Should Be Banned in Civilised Countries. *JAMA* 1983:**249(2)**;250.

11 Casson IR, Siegel O, Sham R, Campbell EA, Tarlau M, DiDomenico A. Brain damage in modern boxers. *JAMA* 1984:**251(20)**;2663-7.

12 Maguire JI, Benson WE. Retinal injury and detachment in boxers. *JAMA* 1986:**255(18)**;2451-3.

13 Jordan BD, Zimmerman RD. Computed tomography and magnetic resonance imaging comparisons in boxers. *JAMA* 1990:**263(12)**;1670-4.

14   Lundberg G D. Boxing should be banned in civilized countries - round 2. *JAMA* 1984:**251(20)**;2696-8.

15   Lundberg GD. Boxing should be banned in civilised countries - round 3. *JAMA* 1986:**255(18)**;2483-5.

16   O'Conner F. Boxing: The Preparticipation Evaluation'. *Military Medicine* 1991:**156(8)**;391.

APPENDIX ONE

Injuries and fatalities in boxing 1985-1993

Injuries and fatalities occurring in boxing — where known, amateurs are highlighted. This list is not intended to be exhaustive and has been compiled from press reports since publication of the 1984 Boxing report, held within the BMA.

1992 Ramon Gomez – American amateur aged 18 – died 18 hours after first practice fight

1991 Jose Malca – Peruvian amateur bantam weight – in a coma for 3 days before dying

1991 Minouru Katsumata – Japanese junior featherweight – died after a coma resulting from a ten round bout

1991 David Ellis – Chilean middleweight – in a coma for 10 days before dying

1991 Kian Kwok Lee – UK amateur welterweight fight – surgery to remove blood clot - required life support

1991 Michael Watson – UK supermiddleweight – persistent neurological damage after brain surgery to remove blood clot and prolonged coma

1991 Frank Bruno – UK professional – detached retina

1990 Gary Mason – UK professional – detached retina

1990 Mark Goult – UK bantamweight – emergency brain surgery – persistent neurological damage

1989 Rod Douglas – UK middleweight – surgery to remove blood clot - retired

1989 R Darko – UK amateur – operated on for brain haemorrhage

1989 Keith Gorton – UK kickboxer – died

1989 J Gilbertson – amateur – operated on for brain haemorrhage

1988 Rico Velazquez – American lightweight aged 22 – died after knock-out in California State title bout - cerebral haemorrhage causing brain swelling

1988 Horace Notice – UK professional heavyweight – British and Commonwealth Champion – detached retina

1987 Joseph Sticklan – UK amateur aged 15 – brain surgery required, died

1986 Steve Watt – Scottish welterweight – brain surgery required, died three days after fight without regaining consciousness

1985 Antonio Harris – UK professional – lost sight in one eye after being allowed to return to ring having previously sustained retinal damage

APPENDIX TWO

National Medical Associations declaring opposition to boxing at the 1991 Annual Representatives Meeting of the British Medical Association

"The undersigned National Medical Associations express the concerns of the medical profession regarding the dangers of boxing and believe that ultimately it should cease to exist. Modern medical technology demonstrates beyond doubt that chronic brain damage is caused by the recurrent blows to the head experienced by all boxers, amateur and professional alike. As long as it is legal to hit an opponent above the neck, there are no safety precautions which can be taken to prevent this damage."

Australia	Bangladesh	Great Britain
Canada	Denmark	Finalnd
Ghana	Ireland	New Zealand
Nigeria	Norway	South Africa

APPENDIX THREE

Published abstracts of original research on boxers carried out since publication of 1984 Boxing Report

Adams CWM and Bruton CJ. The cerebral vasculature in dementia pugilistica. J Neurol, Neurosurg and Psych 1989;52:600-604

The brains of 22 ex-boxers were examined histologically to determine the frequency of recent or old haemorrhage. Four boxers had died from an acute intracerebral bleed — usually soon after a boxing bout. Seven of the other 18 showed evidence of previous perivascular haemorrhage, as detected by Perls' ferrocyanide test for iron, and a similar number showed minor degrees of meningeal or subpial siderosis, consistent with previous meningeal bleeding; cerebellar siderosis was present in six cases. Seventeen of the 22 boxers showed evidence of recent or past haemorrhage. Control material showed an incidence of 11% for perivascular iron deposition and only 4% for minor degrees of meningeal siderosis.

Breton F et al. Event-related potential assessment of attention and the orienting reaction in boxers before and after a fight. Biological Psychology 1990;31:57-71

Boxers' attention and orienting mechanisms were investigated using event-related brain potential recordings, before and after a fight. This study did not reveal any abnormalities of attention or detection processes. However, a slight deficit in the orientating reaction towards stimuli delivered in the right ear, related to a greater number of blows delivered on the left side of the head was observed.

Brooks N et al. A neuropsychological study of active amateur boxers. J Neurol Neurosurg Psych 1987;50:997-1000

Neuropsychological examinations were carried out on 29 amateur boxers and 19 controls matched for age, ethnicity, and education. There was no evidence of significantly impaired performance in the boxers. Within the boxing group, a variety of features of boxing history were examined as possible predictors of cognitive performance (such as number of knock-outs, duration of boxing). No feature was a significant predictor of lower cognitive performance.

Casson IR et al. Brain damage in modern boxers. JAMA 1984;251(20):2663-2667

Eighteen former and active boxers underwent neurological examination, EEG, computed tomographic scan of the brain, and neuropsychological testing. Eighty-seven percent of the professional boxers had definite evidence of brain damage. All the boxers had abnormal results on at least one of the neuropsychological tests. Brain damage is a frequent result of a career in professional boxing.

Drew RH et al. Neuropsychological deficits in active licensed professional boxers. J Clin Psych 1986;42(3):520-525

Young, active, licensed professional boxers (N=19) were found to display a pattern of neuropsychological deficits consistent with the more severe punch drunk syndrome of years past. These deficits resulted in significantly lower test performance than that of control athletes (N=10) matched for race, age and level of education. Tests that showed significant differences between groups include subtests of the Quick Neurological Screening Test, subtests of the Halstead-Reitan Neuropsychological Test Battery, and the Randt Memory Test. Fifteen of the 19 boxers scored in the impaired range of the Reitan Impairment Index, as compared to two of the 10 controls.

Enzenauer RW et al. Boxing-related injuries in the US army, 1980 through 1985. JAMA 1989;261(10):1463-1466

Boxing-related injuries, serious enough to involve hospitalization in US Army hospitals, were studied from 1980 through 1985. On average, there were 67 hospitalizations annually, with the injured spending an average of 5.1 days in bed and 8.9 days disabled, unfit for duty. There was one death from serious head injury and one instance of unilateral blindness from ocular trauma requiring enucleation. Head injuries accounted for 68% of all the injuries and were more common in the younger and presumably less experienced boxers. The advisability of continued promotion of boxing in the military needs to be addressed.

Haglund Y et al. Does Swedish amateur boxing lead to chronic brain damage? 1. A retrospective medical, neurological and personality trait study. Acta Neurol Scand 1990;82:245-252

Sweden banned professional boxing in 1969 and has also considered banning amateur boxing. We therefore analyzed possible chronic brain damage in 47 former amateur boxers who started their careers after the introduction of stricter Swedish amateur boxing rules. The boxers were compared with three control groups — 25 soccer players, 25 track and field athletes and 19 conscripts. All athletes were interviewed about their sports career, medical history and social variables. They then underwent a physical and a neurological examination, including a mini-mental state examination. Personality traits were investigated and related to their platelet monoamine oxidase (MAO) activity in the athletes as well as in the conscripts. No significant differences were found between the groups in any of the physical or neurological examinations. All had a normal mini-mental state examination. Thus, results from these test methods did not reveal any signs of chronic brain damage from Swedish amateur boxing. Neither were any significant differences found with regard to platelet MAO activity, while significant differences were found in some of the social and personality traits variables.

Haglund Y and Bergstrand G. Does Swedish amateur boxing lead to chronic brain damage? 2. A retrospective study with CT and MRI. Acta Neurol Scand 1990;82:297-302

It is well known that professional boxers can develop chronic traumatic encephalopathy (dementia pugilistica) due to repeated head trauma. Beside CT findings indicating cerebral atrophy, the presence of a cavum septum pellucidum has been reported to indicate encephalopathy. CT findings in amateur boxers are not as well documented. The aim of this study was to find out if morphological changes could be demonstrated among former amateur boxers using CT and MRI. Two control groups of soccer players and track and field athletes in the same age-range were used for comparison. No significant differences in the width of the ventricular system, anterior horn index, width of cortical sulci, signs of vermian atrophy, or the occurrence of a cavum septum pellucidum were found between boxers and controls. A cavum septum pellucidum was found more often in the controls than in the boxers and is probably not a sign of earlier head trauma. MRI confirm no more findings than CT in this retrospective study.

Haglund Y and Persson HE. Does Swedish amateur boxing lead to chronic brain damage? 3. A retrospective clinical neurophysiological study. Acta Neurol Scand 1990;82:353-360

The aim of the present study was to investigate possible chronic brain damage due to Swedish amateur boxing. Forty seven former amateur boxers, 22 with many (HM = high-matched) and 25 with few matches (LM = low-matched) during their career were examined and compared with two control groups of 25 soccer players and 25 track and field athletes in the same age-range. No severe EEG abnormality was found. There was a somewhat higher incidence of slight or moderate EEC deviations among HM-(32%, 7/22) and LM-(36%, 9/25) boxers than among soccer players (20%, 5/25) and track and field athletes (12%, 3/25). Brain electric activity mapping (BEAM), brainstem auditory evoked potential (BAEP) and auditory evoked P 300 potential (P 300) did not differ significantly between the groups. No neurophysiological variable was correlated to the number of bouts, number of lost fights or length of boxing career. Thus, no sign of serious chronic brain damage was found among the amateur boxers or the soccer players and the track and field athletes. However, it cannot be excluded that the EEG differences between the groups may be a sign of slight brain dysfunction in some of the amateur boxers.

Heilbronner RL et al. Neuropsychologic test performance in amateur boxers. Am J Sports Med 1991;19(4):376-380

Cognitive functions of 23 amateur boxers were assessed immediately before and after an amateur boxing event. A range of cognitive measures were employed including tasks of verbal, figural, and incidental memory, motor functions, attention and concentration, and information processing speed. Compared to their prefight performance, boxers demonstrated impairments in verbal and incidental memory, but enhanced executive and motor functions postfight. There were no observed differences between winners and losers on any of the measures. The results are compared to other studies that have shown only minor changes in cognitive functions in amateur boxers compared to controls.

Jordan BD and Campbell EA. Acute injuries among professional boxers in New York State: A two-year survey. The Physician and Sportsmedicine 1988;16(1):87-91

Over a two-year period, we reviewed all acute boxing injuries among professional boxers statewide (484 the first year, 422 the second year). During the study period, the boxers fought 3,110 rounds and incurred 376 injuries (262 craniocerebral injuries, 114 other injuries), ie, they incurred 1.2 injuries per 10 rounds fought (0.8 craniocerebral, 0.4 others). Only 4 boxers required immediate neurological evaluation at a hospital after a fight; 1 of the 4 died as a result of bilateral subdural haematomas. Facial lacerations were the most common other type of injury (66 cases). The authors suggest that severe, acute neurological injuries are rare in professional boxing when strict medical supervision is present. However, they caution that their findings should not be used to draw inferences about the development of chronic neurological injuries among professional boxers.

Jordan BD and Zimmerman RD. Magnetic resonance imaging in amateur boxers. Arch Neurol 1988;45:1207-1208

Nine amateur boxers who participated in the 1985 and 1986 New York City Golden Gloves competition underwent detailed neurologic examinations and magnetic resonance imaging (MRI). All nine boxers were medically suspended secondary to a knock-out or excessive head blows. Neurologic examination results and MRI scans were normal in all nine boxers. Failure to detect abnormalities on the MRI scan, by neurologic examination, or both in these amateur boxers may reflect several factors, including a small sample size, the duration between their last bout and neurologic evaluation, and the lower exposure to head trauma among amateur boxers compared with professionals.

Jordan BD and Zimmerman RD. Computed tomography and magnetic resonance imaging comparisons in boxing. JAMA 1990;263(12):1670-1674

The efficacy of computed tomography (CT) and magnetic resonance imaging (MRI) in identifying traumatic injuries of the brain was compared in a referred population of 21 amateur and professional boxers. Three boxers displayed CT scans with equivocal findings that were verified as artefacts by MRI. Eleven boxers had both CT and MRI scans with normal findings, and 7 boxers had both CT and MRI scans with abnormal findings. There were no instances where abnormalities detected on MRI were not detected on CT scans. These included a subdural haematoma, white matter changes, and a focal contusion. Magnetic resonance imaging appears to be the neuroradiodiagnostic test of choice compared with CT.

Levin HS et al. Neurobehavioural functioning and magnetic resonance imaging findings in young boxers. J Neurosurg 1987;67:657-667

In a prospective investigation of neurobehavioural functioning in young boxers, 13 pugilists and 13 matched control subjects underwent tests of attention, information-processing rate, memory and visuomotor coordination and speed. The results disclosed more proficient verbal learning in the control subjects, whereas delayed recall and other measurements of memory did not differ between the two groups. Reaction time was faster in the boxers than in the control subjects, but no other differences in scores between the boxers and the control subjects at the follow-up examination or in the magnitude of improvement from baseline values. Magnetic resonance imaging, which was performed in nine of the boxers, disclosed normal findings.

McLatchie et al. Clinical neurological examination, neuropsychology, electroencephalography and computed tomographic head scanning in active amateur boxers. J Neurol, Neurosurg Psych 1987;50:96-99

Twenty active amateur boxers were studied seeking evidence of neurological dysfunction and, if present, the best method for detecting it. Seven of these boxers had an abnormal clinical neurological examination, eight an abnormal EEG and nine of 15 examined had abnormal neuropsychometry. The CT scan was abnormal in only one. An abnormal clinical examination correlated significantly (p) with an increasing number of fights, and an abnormal EEG with decreasing age (p). In several of the neuropsychometric tests, the boxers were significantly worse than control (p). Neuropsychometry was the best method for detecting neurological dysfunction.

Murelius O and Haglund Y. Does Swedish amateur boxing led to chronic brain damage? 4. A retrospective neuropsychological study. Acta Neurol Scand 1991;83:9-13.

Does Swedish amateur boxing lead to any permanent neuropsychological deficit, caused by chronic brain damage? Fifty Swedish former amateur boxers, 25 soccer players, and 25 track and field athletes were investigated by standardized neuropsychological tests. In only one test did the groups differ significantly. Boxers who had taken part in a large number of bouts had a slightly inferior finger-tapping performance. None of the boxers were considered to have definite signs of intellectual impairment. In conclusion modern Swedish amateur boxing does not seem to lead to significant signs of neuropsychological impairment or "punch drunkenness" (dementia pugilistica), nor does it seem to differ in this respect from soccer playing or track and field sports.

Roberts GW. Immunochemistry of Neurofibrillary Tangles in Dementia Pugilistica and Alzheimer's Disease: Evidence for Common Genesis. Lancet 1988:1456-1457

A battery of antisera that specifically stained the tangles of Alzheimer's disease also stained the tangles in all eight cases of dementia pugilistica (punch drunk syndrome). Since the paired helical filament antigens found in Alzheimer type neurofibrillary degeneration are present in the tangles of dementia pugilistica the pathogenesis of tangle formation in these conditions is likely to be the same; thus head injury may be a predisposing factor or environmental trigger for Alzheimer's disease.

Roberts G W, Allsop D, Bruton C. The occult aftermath of boxing. J Neurol Neurosurg Psych 1990;53:373-378

The repeated head trauma experienced by boxers can lead to the development of dementia pugilistica (DP) — punch drunk syndrome. The neuropathology of DP in a classic report by Corsellis et al describes the presence of numerous neurofibrillary tangles in the absence of plaques, in contrast to the profusion of tangles and plaques seen in Alzheimer's disease (AD). The DP cases used in that report were re-investigated with immunocytochemical methods and an antibody raised to the beta-protein present in AD plaques. We found that all DP cases with substantial tangle formation showed evidence of extensive beta-protein immunoreactive deposits (plaques). These diffuse "plaques" were not visible with Congo-red or standard silver stains. The degree of beta-protein deposition was comparable to that seen in AD. Our data indicate that the present neuropathological description of DP (tangles but no plaques) should be altered to acknowledge the presence of substantial beta-protein deposition (plaques). The molecular markers present in the plaques and tangles of DP are the same as those in AD. Similarities in clinical symptoms, distribution of pathology and neurochemical deficits also exist. Epidemiological studies have shown that head injury is a risk factor in AD. It is probable that DP and AD share common pathogenic mechanisms leading to tangle and plaque formation.

Sabharwal RK et al. Chronic traumatic encephalopathy in boxers. J Assoc Phys India 1987;35(8):571-573

Four Indian boxers developed a progressive neurological disorder. Neuropsychological examination, EEG and computed tomography revealed them to be suffering from chronic traumatic encephalopathy. Boxers should be kept under medical surveillance during their careers and subsequently.

Tokuda T et al. Re-examination of ex-boxers' brains using immuno-histochemistry with antibodies to amyloid beta-protein and tau protein. Acta Neuropathol 1991;82:280-285

A histopathological study was carried out on the brains of eight ex-boxers (ages 56 to 83) using conventional histological staining methods and immunocytochemistry with antibodies to amyloid beta-protein and the PHF-related tau protein. All cases showed a large number of tau-immunoreactive neurofibrillary tangles and also beta-protein immunoreactive senile plaques in the cortex. In the areas with many neurofibrillary tangles, neuropil threads with tau-immunoreactivity were also observed, and some of the senile plaque lesions were surrounded by abnormal neurites with tau-immunoreactivity. Moreover, three cases revealed beta-protein-type cerebrovascular amyloid deposits on both leptomeningeal and cortical blood vessels. The present observations indicate that the cerebral pathology of dementia pugilistica (punch drunk syndrome) is very similar to that of Alzheimer's disease and suggest that these two disorders share some common aetiological and pathogenic mechanisms.

APPENDIX FOUR

Psychiatric, neurological and physiological consequences of head trauma

(Abridged from Roberts GW, Leigh NP, Weinberger D. *Neuropsychiatric disease*. London: Gower Medical Press, 1993.)

Introduction

Blows delivered to the head can cause damage to nerve cells. A single heavy blow or the cumulative effects of a series of lesser blows can result in brain damage sufficient to cause cognitive deficits and behavioural abnormalities as well as neurological symptoms. Damage to blood vessels can cause acute intracranial haematomas that result in death or lifelong disability.

Damage arises from the pure physical effects of trauma (such as swelling and haemorrhage) and from the neurochemical consequences of ischaemia (lack of blood flow) which invariably accompanies physical brain damage. Brain damage following trauma can therefore be viewed as having two phases of pathology: an immediate phase resulting from the physical effects of trauma and an acute-chronic phase caused by the physiological response to the resulting ischaemia.

Many boxers who suffer trauma related brain damage are teenagers or young men in their 20's and if physically or psychiatrically disabled, are likely to require extensive rehabilitation and care within their families or in hospital for many years. In addition, the occurrence of the delayed effects of trauma can lead to neuropsychological deficits, intellectual and/or psychiatric problems, neurological problems and degenerative disease later in life.

Acute effects of trauma

The most common clinical history of the acute effects of trauma consist of the triad of symptoms: alteration of consciousness (momentary dazing to prolonged coma), a period of mental confusion, and amnesic defects.

Consciousness is impaired after all but the slightest impacts in non-penetrating head trauma. Often loss of consciousness is complete and the patient falls to the ground and has no response to stimuli, momentary respiratory arrest, reduced blood pressure, pallor and a loss of corneal reflexes. Contraction of limb muscles followed by flaccid paralysis and loss of tendon reflexes occurs. Consciousness returns after a variable interval (related to the magnitude of the trauma), often accompanied by headache, drowsiness, dizziness, and vomiting. The patient's assessment of the duration of unconsciousness is often overestimated as after recovering the capacity to speak the boxer experiences a phase of disorientation and impaired cognitive function before full consciousness is restored. This phase is enormously variable and dependent on the period of unconsciousness and the degree and type of cerebral injury. After periods of unconsciousness lasting several hours, confusion and disorientation may last for several days or weeks. Where the boxer has experienced a deep and extended period of coma, lasting for a number of days and where permanent brain damage is likely, disturbance of neurological function may last for months. Loss of consciousness is usually more severe when trauma causes the skull to rotate on impact.

The time spent unconscious is a good predictor of prognosis. In general the longer the period of unconsciousness, and the deeper the level of coma, the greater the likelihood that the patient has suffered some degree of brain damage and will suffer neuropsychological and psychiatric sequelae. However, patients with a loss of consciousness lasting several hours can make uneventful recoveries.

Irrespective of the magnitude of trauma which induced the loss of consciousness, on recovery the events immediately pre and post trauma are often not remembered. Establishing the extent of such trauma-related periods of amnesia are clinically useful as prognostic indicators. The time from the moment of injury to the time of resumption of normal continuous memory is known as post traumatic amnesia (PTA). This period includes all periods of unconsciousness and overt confusion and additional periods of confusion of memory. Characteristically the return to normal memory is abrupt, thus many patients can, retrospectively, give an accurate determination for the time of PTA. The time when people begin to speak is often thought to mark the end of unconsciousness however, it is in fact only a step on the way to full consciousness. It is this lag period between speaking and return of full ongoing memory that accounts for the PTA being much longer than the length of unconsciousness.

The time from the moment of injury and the last clear memory from before the trauma the patient can recall is known as retrograde amnesia (RA). The time of RA may prove to be very misleading if it is determined soon after injury. Typically the period may be extensive but shrinks dramatically as the effects of post-traumatic confusion diminish. As a rule, assessment of the RA should not be finalised until the patients PTA has been firmly established. The period of RA is typically short lasting from seconds to a minute in most cases and is considerably shorter than the period of PTA. Longer periods of RA are usually confined to severe cases of brain damage although RA is a much less reliable measure of brain damage than is PTA. Long periods of RA which follow mild trauma are often generated by the patients psychological state.

The length of PTA is the most useful (more so than the period of unconsciousness or confusion) indicator for judging the severity of brain damage and the likely prognosis. The period of PTA is a permanent index and is thus available for clinicians to determine long after the acute effects of the injury have resolved. The length of PTA correlates well with objective measures of brain damage (presence of cognitive impairments, motor disorders, aphasia etc) and with the time that will elapse before the patient returns to work.

Post-traumatic coma may be deep from the beginning or may deteriorate in the immediate aftermath of the trauma due to oedema and/or intracranial haemorrhage. Surgical intervention to evacuate blood from inside the skull is indicated when comatose patients show signs of brainstem compression such as failing respiration, falling blood pressure and fixed dilated pupils. Investigations by CT and MRI greatly facilitate the assessment of primary brain damage and the presence of secondary brain damage due to blood clot, brain swelling or hypoxic brain damage.

Neurological sequelae

Lesions of the cranial nerves are commonly seen (eg loss of sense of smell, visual field defects, ocular palsies) after head trauma, as are motor disorders resulting from cortical and brain stem lesions. Complications arising from intracranial bleeding are likely to give rise to focal neurological damage related to the area of brain damaged.

Epilepsy is one of the commonest chronic neurological sequelae, and can be classed as early epilepsy (during the first week after injury) or late epilepsy (developing after a delay of months). Early epilepsy rarely occurs in the absence of prolonged PTA, depressed fracture of the skull or intracranial bleeding. The occurrence of early epilepsy considerably enhances the risk of late epilepsy. In late epilepsy the first fit occurs 12 months or more after the trauma in 50% of patients. Late epilepsy is the most frequent delayed complication of a non-penetrating head injury. The risk is greater in patients who had an intracranial haematoma, a compound depressed fracture, early epilepsy, focal brain damage and, focal brain damage with prolonged unconsciousness. The close relationship between the degree of focal brain damage and the risk of post-traumatic epilepsy implies that direct destruction of brain tissue is the most important cause of post-traumatic epilepsy in any type of head injury.

Progressive Neurodegeneration — punch drunk syndrome (Dementia Pugilistica)

Large numbers of concussive or subconcussive blows to the head, in professional boxers for example, result in the occurrence of minor brain damage. Areas of hypoperfusion in the brain have been demonstrated in amateur boxers using SPECT imaging. CT and MRI studies have demonstrated focal abnormalities, ventricular enlargement and cortical atrophy consistent with a more chronic process in professional fighters. Continual minor brain damage can lead to the accumulation of neurological signs and induce a progressive neurodegenerative syndrome. This condition, known as dementia pugilistica or the punch drunk syndrome, becomes clinically obvious years after the last fight and can be described in three stages:

Stage 1   affective disorder, mild incoordination

Stage 2   dysphasia, apraxia, agnosia, apathy, blunting of affect and neurological signs

Stage 3   global cognitive decline and parkinsonism

The syndrome is present in about 20% of older professional boxers (50 years)[1] and is more likely to develop in boxers with long careers who have been dazed if not knocked out on many occasions. The brains of these patients have a characteristic pattern of brain damage, the principal features of which are, fenestrated septum, degeneration of the substantia nigra, neuronal loss in cortex and cerebellum, cortical neurofibrillary tangle formation and, cortical diffuse beta-amyloid plaques.

The molecular pathology of the punch drunk syndrome appears to be very similar to that seen in Alzheimer's disease. These observations have been used to argue that severe or repeated head trauma can trigger Alzheimer's disease.

Haemorrhage

Intracranial haemorrhages are the commonest cause of clinical deterioration and death in patients who have experienced a lucid interval after their injury. The risk of such haemorrhages can turn even an apparently trivial head injury into a life threatening condition. After a head injury haemorrhages can occur into the extradural, subdural or subarachnoid spaces, the brain itself (intracerebral) and the ventricles of the brain.

Extradural, subdural and intracerebral haematomas cause expanding intracranial lesions which increase intracranial pressure and compress the surface of the brain. Prompt surgical intervention to evacuate the blood can relieve these conditions. Post-traumatic subarachnoid haemorrhage is often associated with contusions and intraventricular haemorrhage and occasionally a late effect may be normal pressure hydrocephalus.

Contusion

Contusions are a form of bruising of the brain and are a characteristic pathology seen in boxers. Contusions are thought to be a product of the external (injury-causing) force applied to the head and the inertia of the brain inside the skull. Next to the contusion there is a zone of vessels which have been physically disrupted and show increased capillary permeability together with a loss of normal physiological regulation. This disruption allows water to enter the area causing local oedema.

Diffuse brain damage

Loss of consciousness or loss of neurological function can occur seconds after a head injury. It is thought that this sudden loss of function and a great deal of the chronic neurological damage is due to the diffuse brain damage which occurs at multiple sites throughout the brain. Neuropathology has defined four main types of diffuse brain damage which arise at the moment of injury or which develop as a slow response to the trauma: diffuse axonal injury, diffuse vascular injury, raised intracranial pressure and brain swelling, and, ischaemia.

Diffuse axonal injury/diffuse vascular injury

Patients who sustain severe diffuse axonal injury are unconscious from the moment of impact, do not experience a lucid interval and remain unconscious, vegetative or at least severely disabled until death. The clinical picture has been described as primary brain stem injury. Diffuse vascular damage can be described as the occurrence of many small haemorrhages scattered throughout the brain and is another common consequence of head injury.

Raised intracranial pressure and brain swelling

The volume of the skull is finite. When expanding mass lesions occur (eg haematoma) surplus volume within the cranial vault is filled and regions of the brain are compressed to accommodate the lesion. This ability for 'spatial compensation' is limited and once it is exceeded intracranial pressure begins to rise. When pressure begins to exceed the upper range of normal for minutes at a time brain damage may occur.

Brain swelling often occurs in addition to vascular damage and is a major factor contributing to an increase in intracranial pressure (along with haemorrhages). Brain swelling is thought to be caused in two ways; by cerebral vasodilatation and an increase in cerebral blood volume (ie. congestive brain swelling) or by an increase in the water content of neuronal tissue (ie cerebral oedema). The delayed clinical deterioration (2-3 days after injury) in patients with a subdural haematoma is more likely to be caused by brain swelling and a subsequent increase in intracranial pressure than enlargement of the haematoma itself. CT and MRI can give reliable indications of raised intracranial pressure and also indicate the site of the problem.

Ischaemia

The human brain has a high metabolic rate and as a result the volume of blood flow is extensive. Different cognitive tasks result in altered patterns of blood flow. Cerebral blood vessels alter their diameter (autoregulation) in at least two ways in response to physiological stimuli thus ensuring that additional metabolic demand is met and the pattern of blood flow is controlled. These responses ensure an even blood flow which remains almost constant between arterial pressures of 60-150 mmHg. The existence of these complicated and sensitive regulatory mechanisms enables the brain to orchestrate its metabolic activity in a dynamic fashion and respond to changing demand within seconds. Such sensitivity explains the catastrophic effects of arbitrary disruptions in the brains blood supply which might last for minutes or hours due to trauma.

The degree of damage caused by ischaemia is related to the magnitude of the reduction in blood flow and the period of reduced blood flow. The interplay between these parameters is obviously complicated and is made more so by the fact that different classes of neurones within the brain have differing vulnerabilities to ischaemic damage. The onset of ischaemia induces a cascade of molecular events and it is likely that one or more of these events may directly trigger neuronal destruction or reduce the neurones' capacity to survive. Recent studies show that once initiated, such mechanisms can lead inexorably to cell death independent of the degree or presence of ischaemia.

Psychiatric symptoms

The range of psychiatric symptoms which occur as a consequence of head trauma is wide and includes, phobias, anxiety states, depression, neurotic disorders and, cognitive deficits. These problems are clinically important as difficulty in obtaining employment and problems due to interpersonal or social interaction are more likely to be caused by psychiatric symptoms than by physical handicap.

Post traumatic syndrome is characterised by the presence of persistent headache, dizziness and to a greater or lesser extent fatigue, insomnia, poor memory, irritability and emotional lability. However, the exact nature and even the existence of the syndrome has been the subject of debate. The symptoms often persist for months after the traumatic event and are often observed to be aggravated by stress, tension or depression. In many cases the symptoms lack clear precipitants and are very resistant to treatment. The post-traumatic syndrome is rare in the presence of trauma which causes intellectual impairment or neurological disability.

References

1   Roberts AM. *Brain damage in boxers. A study of prevalence of traumatic encephalopathy among ex-professional boxers.* London: Pitman, 1969.

APPENDIX FIVE

Clinical Questionnaire

Investigation into brain damage sustained by boxing

IDENTIFICATION

Patient's Initials: _____ Identification Number: _____
(not essential)

Name of Reporting Doctor: _____

Patient's Age *(yrs)*: _____ Occupation: _____

SUMMARY OF BOXING CAREER *(Note: Referee stopping fight because of injury to patient, equivalent to K.O.)*

Schoolboy Career:

Age commenced *(yrs)*: _____ Age retired *(yrs)*: _____

No of bouts: _____ Wins: _____

Losses: _____

K.O.'s sustained: _____

Amateur Career:

Age commenced *(yrs)*: _____ Age retired *(yrs)*: _____

Weight category: _____

No of bouts: _____ Wins: _____

Losses: _____ K.O's sustained: _____

APPENDIX FIVE

Level Achieved: *(please tick appropriate boxes)*

   (i) Novice: ☐   National: ☐
   (ii) Intermediate: International:
   (iii) Senior:
   (iv) Championship:

Professional Career:

Age commenced *(yrs)*:_____ Age retired *(yrs)*:_____

Weight category: _____

No of bouts: _____ Wins: _____

                                                             Losses: _____

                                                             K.O.s sustained: _____

List of championships held: _____

_____

_____

Unlicensed Career: (if known)

Comments:_____

_____

_____

_____

MEDICAL CONDITION

Approximate date of onset:_____

Presenting symptom:_____

Symptoms present when seen:
(please tick apropriate box depending on degree of severity + = mild, +++ = severe)

+ ++ +++

1. Depression
2. Personality change *(specify)*

3. Memory problems
4. Intellectual loss
5. Dysarthria
6. Clumsiness
7. Tremor
8. Other Extrapyramidal symptoms
9. Weakness
10. Headaches
11. Giddiness or vertigo
12. Epilepsy
13. Others *(specify)*

Neurological signs when seen: *(please tick appropriate box)*

+ ++ +++

1. Dementia
2. Memory loss:
    Type *(specify)*

3. Depression
4. Personality disorder
5. Dysarthria
6. Nystagmus
7 Oculomotor disorder
8. Ataxia
9. Parkinsonian signs:
    Tremor
    Rigidity
    Posture
    Poverty of movement
10. Pyramidal signs
11. Visual defects
12. Deafness
13. Sensory changes
14. Disordered gait
15. Others *(specify)*

APPENDIX FIVE

Additional Medical Disorders: *(if any)*

	+	++	+++
1. Cerebrovascular disease			
2. Hypertension			
3. Alcohol abuse			
4. Drug abuse			
5. Psychosexual			
6. Others (specify)			

_____

Course of Symptoms: *(brief description)*_____

_____

_____

_____

_____

Investigation: *(summarise reports)*

1. EEG Recording: _____

_____

_____

_____

2. CT Scan _____

_____

_____

_____

3. MRI Scan _____

_____

_____

_____

BRITISH MEDICAL ASSOCIATION

4. Others _____ _____

Diagnosis: _____

Outcome if known: _____

Additional comments: _____

Thank you for taking the time to complete this questionnaire

Please return to:

Sallie Robins
Scientific Affairs
British Medical Association
BMA House
Tavistoci Square
LONDON WC1H 9JP

Tel: 071 383 6225
Fax: 071 383 6233

Index

Index

D

E

F

G

H

I

L

M

N

O

P

功夫

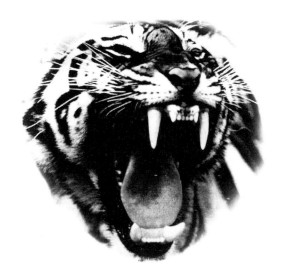

虎

This book is dedicated to Daphne Pearl Green, Lucan Green, Hazel Davis, Vincent Davis and all the students of MD Martial Arts.

Keep the spirit of the tiger within you always.

Sifu Marc Davis

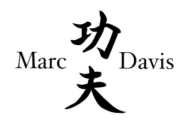

Marc Davis

M.D. MARTIAL ARTS

For All Serious Martial Artists

The Scientific Approach

First published in 2005 by MD Martial Arts

Marc Davis
255 Melfort Road
Thornton Heath
Surrey CR7 7RW

© Marc Davis 2005
email: mdmartialarts@yahoo.co.uk
www.md-martialarts.com
Primary Mobile number 07960599125
Secondary Mobile Number 07957378530

British Library Cataloguing in Publication Data
A CIP record for this book is available from the British Library.

ISBN 0-9549573-0-X
Cover, text design and production of book by Richard Reid/Novel Graphic.

Contents

ᵢⱼ

About the Author

Sifu Marc Davis was born in England in 1974 and spent the early years of his life growing up in Jamaica. He was always a very physical person and at the age of six years old he had his first introduction to martial arts in the form of boxing and karate by his family as his uncle and many of his cousins are martial artist. 3 years later he walked in to his first martial arts school at the age of 9 years old. In his own words he knew this was something that he would do for the rest of his life. Destiny!

Sifu marc has been practicing and studying the martial arts for 23 years, this has included many different styles.

1) shukukai karate
2) Renshinkai karate
3) Freestyle kung fu
4) wado ryu karate
5) Aikido
6) Boxing
7) Kickboxing
8) Wing Chun kung fu
9) Wu shu Kwan
10) Pencak silat
11) Yang style tai chi
12) Chi gong – internal breathing
13) Chen style tai chi
14) M. D martial arts

He has also study holistic arts such as yoga and continues to practice his martial arts with even greater desire and dedication after all these years remaining open minded and always willing to learn. After gaining a very strong foundation and studying many different styles he still felt unfulfilled and knew that something was missing. With his burning desire to be the best he developed his own unique system of martial arts known as md martial arts, he felt that his name best respresented his art as it was based on himself his own experiences within the martial arts and also his life, and ultimately his self expression.

Safety

Safety (following the proper procedures)

The author and the publishers do not accept any responsibility for any injuries that may occur to persons whilst following the exercises and techniques described in this book.

The author strongly advises anyone interested in practising martial arts on any level, mentally, physically or spiritually, to first seek the advice of a doctor and train under the guidance of a fully qualified instructor.

History of Martial Arts

In the history of warfare whether it be cavemen, gladiators or modern armies some form of combat has been present throughout the history of the world.

The term martial arts roughly translated from the chinese term Wu Shu, means 'good effort'. The specific skills of martial arts whether with empty hands or with the use of weapons can be traced back as far as 1500 years.

China and India are the two main countries credited with the development of martial arts and bringing it to the masses. As the story goes a Buddhist monk by the name of Buddadharma was an expert in different methods of breathing and meditation, he travelled to the shaolin temple in china where the monks were highly skilled in hand to hand combat as well as the use of weapons. Upon arriving, he saw that they were in need of spiritual training to strengthen the mind, along with deep breathing and exercises that would strengthen their bodies not only externally but also internally. These methods are what we now know as chi gung breathing and exercise. This completed the monks physically, mentally and spiritually, making them complete warriors and martial artists of the highest level. The shaolin temple is still considered the birthplace of martial arts and its monks are regarded as the best in the world.

There are many different forms and styles of martial arts, hundreds in fact, that cover all the different areas of combat such as the four ranges – long, medium, close and grappling. These styles also cover striking that utilises every part of the body – fist, elbows, knee, feet, head and the palms to name but a few. These arts also include joint locks, chokes, throws, pressure points and weapons, along with the previously mentioned physical exercises, internal breathing and meditation.

In the beginning most of these styles were developed by watching different animals fight and mimicking their movements. Opposite is a list of some of the most popular styles taught in china.

wu shu

good effort

Tiger
Eagle claw
Snake
Mantis
Dragon
Crane
Monkey

Phoenix
Leopard
Tai chi
Bua gua
Hsing I
Wing chun
Chin na
Choy li fat
Hung gar
Pak mei
Shaolin

*Be positive
but not
arrogant and
you will
perform to
the best of
your
abilities.'*

Marc Davis

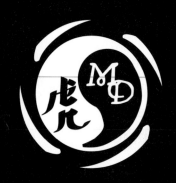

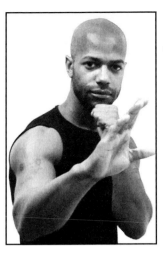

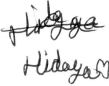

History of MD Martial Arts

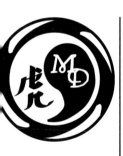

The system of M.D Martial Arts was developed in 1992 by Sifu Marc Davis, the letters MD are the initials of the founder of the system – Marc Davis, and represent his development within martial arts and his unique expression of the knowledge gained on this journey.

This system is based on experience of the many different styles studied by Sifu Marc Davis, with a strong influence from Chinese Kung Fu. He developed this system with an emphasis on modern-day combat and self-defence.

The system initially came about from Sifu Marc Davis' desire to be proficient in all areas and ranges of martial arts, in order to be a complete martial artist. He wanted to develop not just an art form, or sport, but a system that would be useful in real life situations. He also demanded that this not be a static

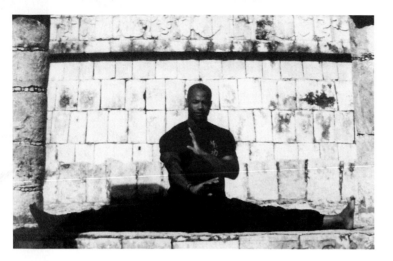

'you will achieve clarity of thought when you posses a clear and peaceful mind'

Marc Davis

system, but one which develops with each individual and over time.

To date Sifu Marc Davis has taught over 500 students across England and around the world, ranging from people who have never trained in martial arts to people who are black belts in other disciplines and people involved in security and bodyguard work. This in itself speaks volumes for the M.D system, with its unique, direct and effective approach.

The Aim of
Martial Arts

The aim of martial arts may vary in many ways from person to person, and people study and practice for many different reasons.

For example, people may study martial arts to boost their self-confidence, to improve their fitness, as a sport, to compete, and even to socialise. In my view, the aim of martial arts is a journey of self-discovery, finding out who you are and what your physical, mental and spiritual capabilities are. It also teaches etiquette, discipline and respect for yourself and others.

Martial arts is much more than just fighting, you learn to use your body in different ways in order to express yourself, much like a musician expressing themselves through their instrument. Our instrument is our body and through this we learn to develop ourselves, ultimately facing our fears, achieving our goals and becoming a better person.

The Link between Animals and the Arts

Since the beginning of martial arts animals have played a vital role in the development of many of the traditional martial arts.

Techniques and styles have been based on the characteristics and movements of specific animals. Examples include the Snake, Crane, Mantis, Monkey, Eagle, Tiger, Leopard, and Dragon. Although the dragon is a mythical creature it holds a very strong place in Chinese culture. These animal styles, as they are known, were developed from studying the movements of various different animals – particularly when in combat with each other.

The following are examples of traits specific to certain animals that have been adapted to develop some of the traditional martial arts systems:

Snake – fast and direct

Crane – evasive and deceptive

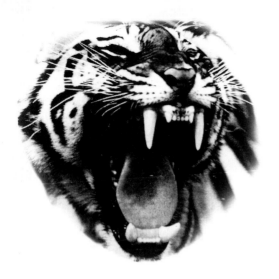

Mantis – powerful grip

Monkey – elusive and deceptive

Eagle – strong claws, powerful grip and awareness

Tiger – agile and aggressive

Dragon – powerful and mystical.

'He who knows men is clever, he who knows himself has insight, he who conquers men has force, he who conquers himself is truly strong

Lao Tze

The traits and characteristics of these animals were used in combination with the mechanics of the human body to develop strikes and techniques such as punching, kicking, throwing and joint locks. This combined with the right state of mind to mimic the animals and created the animal styles we know today.

Different Styles of Martial Arts

China

Tiger
Snake
Crane
Monkey
Dragon
Eagle
Mantis
Wing Chun
Pak Mei
Tai Chi
Hsing Hi
Bua Qua
Choy Li Fut
Hung gar
go-ti
Shaolin

Japan

Iaido
Aiilido
Kenjitsu
Kendo
Ninjitsu
Judo
Wado Ryu
Shotokaw
Shokukai
Kyokushinkai
Gojo Ryu

India

Piak
Philipines
Escrima
Kali
Dumog

Thailand

Thai Boxing
Krabi Krabon

Greece

Pankration
Roman Wrestling
Mu-tau

Russia

Sambo

Korea

Taewondo
Mu Kendo
Kuk Sool Won
Hwarawg-do
Hapkido

Indonesia

Pencak Silat
Gulat wrestling
Baru Silat
Harimau Silat

功夫

Preparing the Body

It is very important to prepare the body for training irrespective of how basic or advanced your training session will be. There are two major reasons for preparing the body; the first and most important is to avoid injuries to your muscles, ligaments and bones. The second reason is to help prepare the mind for the task ahead.

There are three major stages of preparing the body:

Loosening the joints – neck, shoulders, wrists, waist, knees and ankles.

Warm up – to warm the muscles and protect them from injury. This can be done using any form of cardiovascular exercise, e.g. jogging, jump jacks or shuttle runs. Equipment may also be used, e.g. skipping, pad work, bag work and cycling.

Stretching – this is done as a final preparation to avoid muscle injury and to improve flexibility. The major muscle groups that need to be stretched are the

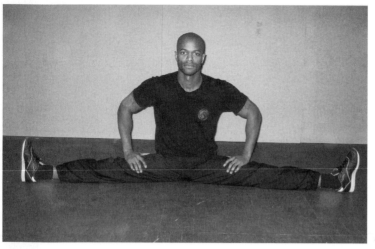

Box splits
(Adductors and groin stretch)

shoulders and deltoids, triceps, forearms, quadriceps, hamstrings, groin adductor (inner thigh), abductor (outer thigh) and calf muscles. Below are some pictures to show you the correct way to stretch. As the upper body stretches are quite basic we will focus on the advanced leg stretches as the leg muscles are much harder to improve flexibility and are also more susceptible to injury. Each stretch should be held for a minimum of 30 seconds; the maximum is dependent on the individual's level of flexibility and the duration you intend to train for.

'remember the will to try is the will to succeed. Everything comes to you when you are ready and worthy to receive it'

Marc Davis

Hamstring stretch

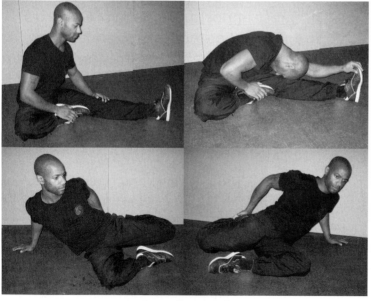

Quad stretch

These also gently stretch the upper body.

Preparing the Mind

As mentioned in the previous chapter, by preparing the body the mind begins to focus and prepare itself on a basic level.

However, to fully prepare the mind - to be alert, calm, passive, but ready to respond - there are major exercises and drills to perform with endless variations. The following are the most used techniques to prepare the mind.

Meditation

Concentrate on images with your eyes closed, focus on yourself and your technique. Meditation can also be done with your eyes open by focusing on an object, for example the flame of a candle. Anything where you have to maintain concentration and not allow yourself to be distracted by mundane thoughts is a form of meditation.

Deep Breathing

This helps to focus the mind whilst relaxing and

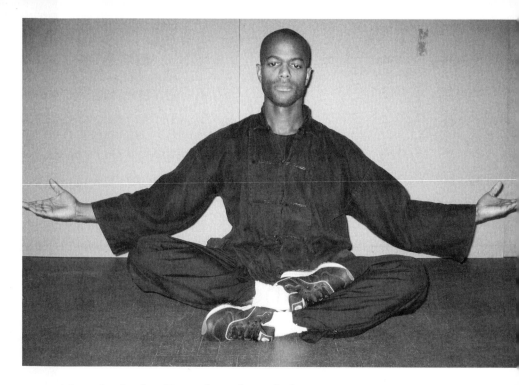

energising the body. Deep breathing helps to connect
the mind and body preparing you for the training
ahead whether it be individual training, a martial arts
class, practising techniques or sparring.

*'If you hav
negative
thoughts
about
combat
don't both
turning up
There is n
place for
such
thoughts'*

Marc Davis

Determination and Will Power

In all aspects of life we all have our goals and things that we would like to achieve. The possibilities are endless regardless of what you wish to achieve and in what field. In the world of martial arts, this is no different.

Once you have found the style that best suits you and a good teacher, it is important to know what it is that you expect to gain from your martial arts training. Your goal may be self defence, strength, flexibility, balance, coordination, confidence, improved memory, improved circulation or general health and fitness. The potential reasons for training are endless but as a whole martial arts is a way of life. It will develop you completely, physically mentally and spiritually. The question is what level you wish to attain and how hard are you prepared to work for it. This is where your dedication, determination and will power come in.

Throughout the journey of your training your will

power will become stronger and your determination greater as you strive towards your goals. Remember, patience is essential, as frustration will consume you when the going gets tough. You may find the physical demands too great on the body and mind, or find certain techniques difficult to understand and apply physically. Be patient and remember why you are doing this and what your ultimate goals are. With the development of your training your mind and body will continue to develop also. It is during these times that your will power will grow and become stronger; you will then be able to see your goals clearly and have the determination and desire to achieve them. The only boundary to what you can achieve is yourself.

'If people have no faith I don know wha they are good for, can a vehicle travel without a link to a source of power'

Confuscius

'Learn to be patient and good things will come to you'

Marc Davis

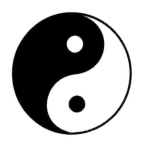

Principles and Philosophy

There are many different forms of philosophy and principles, but one of the most well known is that of the Chinese and Japanese cultures, a way of life: yin and yang. Yin and Yang is represented by a circle, half black and half white with each half containing a small circle of the opposite colour. This symbol of yin and yang represents duality and totality, two forces or energies coexisting in perfect balance and harmony.

The white section of the circle represents – female / day / cold / softness. The black section represents the opposite – male / night / warmth / firmness.

As they both contain a part of each other they maintain perfect unity.

Anything that moves towards the extreme will not last and will ultimately destroy itself. However, at the same

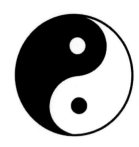

time not to strive is not to succeed: you must find a happy medium.

For example, it is like the tree that stands in the mist of a strong wind; if it is too soft it will simply be uprooted and blown away, too rigid and it will break. But the tree that is firm but soft, strong but flexible, is able to yield with the wind and retain its firm root in the ground demonstrates a perfect balance of yin and yang.

It is important to note that the yin and yang philosophy has many more applications than martial arts. It is a way of life for many, particularly in the Chinese culture. The Chinese use yin and yang in all aspects of their life, but most commonly in martial arts, their cuisine and, most importantly, their health. Chinese medicine and acupuncture is based on the principles of yin and yang. If a person is ill the doctor will treat them according to their lack of or excessive chi. This is ultimately an imbalance: too much or not enough yin or yang. The correct balance of yin and yang makes the person better and enables them to lead a much healthier life.

'to find your medium is to find perfect harmony in your life'

Marc Davi

Traditional Martial Arts

Traditional Martial Arts are the basis from which all martial art forms have evolved.

This is martial arts in its purest form, undiluted, containing set movements, katas forms and pre-arranged movements that contain all the techniques of the style. This is the way in which traditional martial arts are taught from master to student and from generation to generation. This is not to say that traditional martial arts are set in their ways; they are always adaptable but stay true to their heritage and tradition. The following are some of the key aspects of traditional training:

– *Techniques are performed in lines.*

– *Conditioning of the body – this is done by striking certain areas of the body, for example forearms and shins, in order to strengthen them. This can by done on your own, with equipment or with a partner.*

– *Board and brick breaking.*

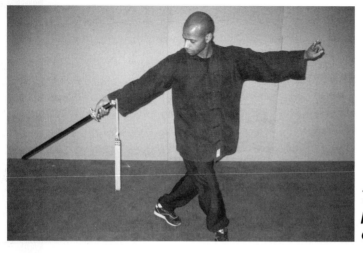

The author practicing Tai chi chuan sword form

— *Following move for move the techniques that the master performs.*

— *Repetition of techniques and katas to train the mind and body and develop power, speed and accuracy.*

— *The meaning and application of katas.*

— *Weapons: most of which are not useful for modern day combat, for example sai, long staff, three section staff, and katana.*

— *Muscle development gained not by weights, but by using resistance from your own body or from a partner.*

'never give up, the body may be weak but the spirit can overcome anything'

Marc Davis

Modern Martial Arts

What is modern martial arts?

It is a system or style that was developed fairly recently unlike traditional martial arts which was developed hundreds or thousands of years ago. Like most things, Martial Arts has been evolving since its very beginning.

Styles that are more functional in today's modern world evolve through the practicioners quest for perfection and to adapt to change. Training can be just as hard but modern equipment such as punch bags and weights now help modern martial artists hone their body and techniques. The use of padding and protective clothing for sparring and even training to music are other examples of modern martial art practices.

Some teachers of the martial arts discard many of the traditional training methods but retain the etiqutte of discipline, respect, loyalty etc.

It is important to remember that, for all the

'expression of art is ultimately the expression of self'

differences between traditional and modern martial arts, the quest for black belt or to reach a senior level **Marc Davis**

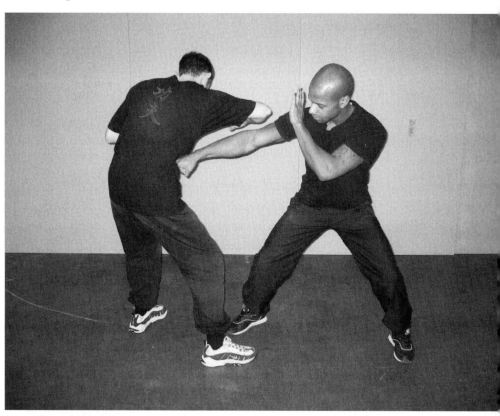

is ultimately the mastery of your chosen style and self.

The Four Ranges of Martial Arts

The fighting ranges.

Within the martial arts there are different ranges or distances, from which to perform techniques. It is important to note that each style of martial arts specialises in one or two of the four ranges, thus having a weakness in the others and ultimately an incomplete style/system.

There are four ranges in total and we will look at them individually in this chapter.

The first range of fighting is long; in combat the legs normally dictate this fighting distance unless weapons are used. The following are some of the most common kicks, regardless of whether the style is from China, Japan, Korea, India or the Philippines:

Front kick
Back kick
Roundhouse
Side
Hook

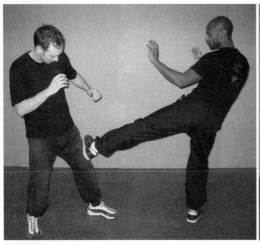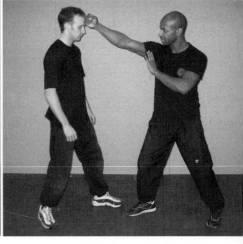

1 – The First Range - Long   *2 – The Second Range - Mediu*

The second range in combat is medium range; this can also utilise the legs but only using short kicks. The most common weapons are the arms, which would be almost fully extended. This then involves striking with various parts of the hands. These parts include a closed fist, open hands using the fingers, palm, edge of hand and even the wrist. Below are some examples:

> Jab
> Rear cross
> Palm hand
> Heel strike
> Finger jab.

The third range is close; this involves all weapons of the body utilising very short fighting techniques such as:

> Hooks
> Uppercut
> Elbows
> Head butts
> Knees
> Takedowns
> Sweeps.

The fourth and final range is grappling; once again this is a close range skill, but it differs from the

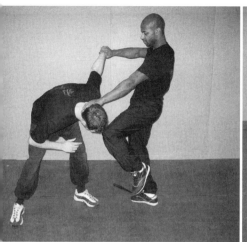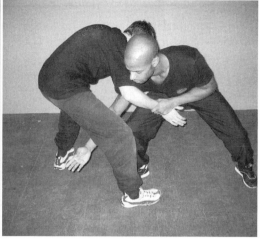

– The Third Range - Close   4 – The Fourth Range - Grappling

previous close range as it makes less use of striking and places more emphasis on restraining techniques such as joint locks and chokes. Skills like throws, sweeps and breaking techniques are also utilised. These techniques can all be performed from a standing position or on the ground.

Weapons – Traditional and Modern

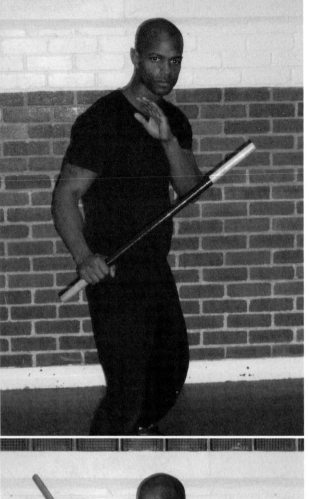

1 Single Short Stick commonly known as Kali Sticks. Most famously used in Phillipino martial Arts.

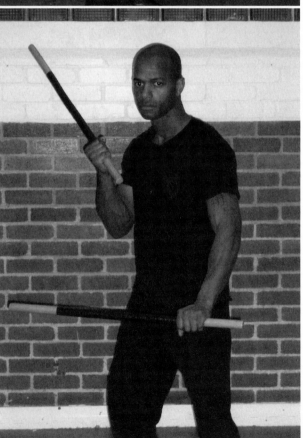

2 Double Sticks

The methods for using the single or double sticks vary from using the long section to strike, the short section and the point, as well as aplying locks, throws and chokes.

Double bladed
nife. Used
specificaly for close
range combat.
echniques can be
one with either
de of the blade, the
oint or the handle
f the knife.

The Tai chi Sword.
nlike many swords
e major techique
ith this sword is to
e the point.

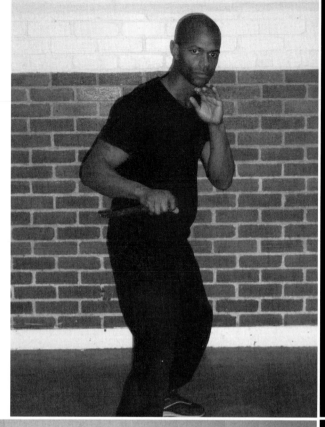

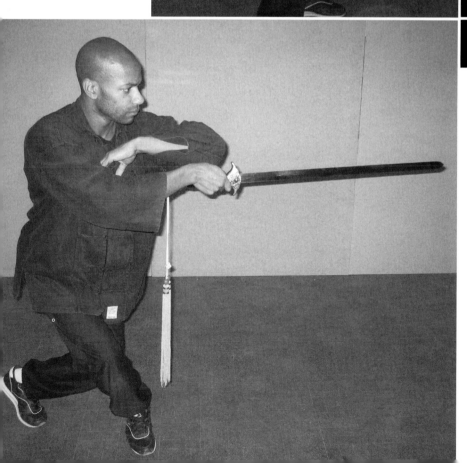

虎

My Opinion on Martial Arts

It is my honest belief that the martial arts are a vehicle through which you can achieve your true potential as a human being. Martial arts teaches you to be disciplined, dedicated, respectful and focused in order to achieve your goals or to overcome any obstacle in your life.

I feel that it is therefore the duty of all teachers/instructors of the martial arts to continue to teach the true essence and code of these arts in order to preserve them for generation to generation.

I write these words with sincerity as I feel we are in danger of losing the pure and real martial arts – the code, the true techniques and the spirit of these arts.

If we look around the hard work and life long journey to achieve mastery has been replaced by weaker versions of the original styles which in turn leads to a lack of understanding of the different styles and poor techniques.

The martial arts were developed in times of war, but now almost everything is sport martial arts, people fighting for medals, trophies and money. There is also the emergence of mixed martial arts, which on a positive note has made most martial artists aware that they need to be skillful in all ranges of combat. On the negative side many people do not have a strong foundation in one core style and become a jack of all trades, but master of none. Instead of seeking proficiency in all areas and achieving fluid techniques in the different art forms, we see wild techniques and punch-ups, with victory often going to the bigger, stronger fighter. This is not the way of the warrior, real martial arts overcomes size and strength with good technique and knowledge. Ultimately there are no rules to limit our options.

ultimately there are no rules to limit our options

External and Internal Style

In the world of martial arts there are many different forms of combat and each has their particular strengths and weaknesses. However, regardless of style there is often one of two categories that they fall into, and that is external or internal.

In this chapter we will look at some of the key points that distinguish the external and internal styles.

It is important for me to state that to some degree all styles contain some basic elements of external martial arts, regardless of where the style is from. If the style emphasises: Brute force or power; excessive large movements; extreme rigidity of the muscles and joints; more direct movements in defence, then these particular styles are gauged more towards the external form of martial arts.

The stronger you are on a physical level is of extreme importance, in order to apply not all, but some of the techniques – in short, to see these styles in motion, they are very effective and visually powerful, based on

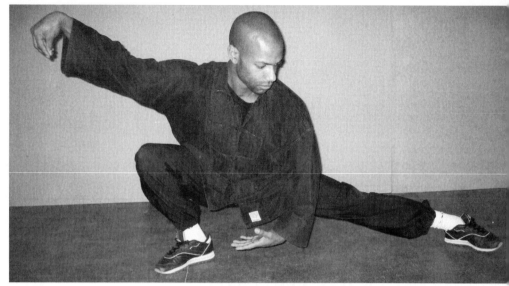

great muscular power and technique, which if faced with an even bigger or stronger opponent may cause problems, for example, some of these techniques will be less effective.

The key points that distinguish the internal style of martial arts: greater emphasis on breathing; small movements in techniques; relaxed muscles; angles/evasive movements in defence; and yielding to the opponent's force.

These internal styles are based on much smaller movements and more sophisticated techniques that often appeal to people who are not physically strong or physically imposing. To see these internal styles in motion, you will appreciate their effectiveness, but on first impressions, it does not seem as powerful as the external styles. This is a common misconception in the world of martial arts in fact the internal styles of martial arts possess true power on every level, physically, mentally and spiritually. It is on these levels that the internal martial arts excel.

Look deeper and you will see the inner workings of all the key points mentioned above in the internal styles with a higher level of sophistication than most other styles, and a deeper understanding of techniques.

36

I must stress that this chapter is not about which method is better, but rather what you want out of martial arts, which method may suit you best as a person physically and mentally.

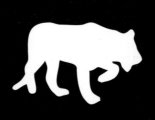

The Code of Martial Arts

In this chapter we will be covering an extremely important aspect of training, which if not understood will affect you in achieving the higher levels within the martial arts.

I am referring to the code of martial arts:

Discipline
Respect
Loyalty
Dedication

The shaolin monks of China or the Samurai warrior of Japan all followed these codes, as should all serious martial artist today. The practice of real martial arts is not a sport or a hobby but rather a way of life, in order to discover oneself.

Now let's look at each of these codes and see why they are so important, and why they can be of great use to your martial arts practice and even your whole way of living.

Discipline & Dedication

In martial arts if you have the right discipline and dedication, you have the right attitude. This will help you build your willpower, which you will need in order to be prepared for the hard training and sacrifices that you will have to make, for example being hurt while sparring or just the pain you feel from performing techniques over and over again. With discipline and the required dedication comes patience and understanding which in turn will lead to many great things.

Respect & Loyalty

It is very important to have respect and loyalty in various different areas within the martial arts especially for your teacher and your chosen style.

With the respect and loyalty you have for your teacher comes great belief, respect in yourself.

Without the above keys in training true progression is not possible, at least not on a higher level.

Finally, these codes within your martial arts manifest themselves in your everyday life making you a better person. For example respect for yourself and for other people will ultimately make you a kinder, more positive, dedicated person with clear morals and principles.

'adaptibility is the way o true under- standing both in martial arts and life, but always be true to who you are.'

Marc Davis

The Best Style

In the world of martial arts there are so many different styles and forms that the inevitable question will arise – what style is the best?

I honestly believe that there is no such thing as the best style. Why? Because I think it is ultimately down to the practitioner, physically, mentally and spiritually. If you understand combat and make sure that your training is as realistic as possible, covering all the ranges it is then simply about being first making sure that you are superior in every way, i.e. speed, power, accuracy, conditioning, mental strength and knowledge. These qualities should then go hand in hand with strategys. It is like two identical instruments made by the same person: if the same person plays them, they sound the same but if different people were to play them the sound would be very different. This is the same when two people express their different styles or the same style of martial arts, their individual interpretation will create inevitable differences.

Every style of martial arts has something to offer and each has positives and negatives. Find a good teacher, practice hard and always be open minded so that you can adapt to any situation. As time passes you will change and grow with your teacher as will your abilities, skill and knowledge. You will progress to a higher level making your chosen style fully functional and effective.

Remember – only you can make your style come alive.

remember – only you can make your style come alive

Mind Frame

The mind is our most important attribute and in everything we do the mind has to be prepared, alert and focused on the job at hand. While training in the martial arts, privately or in a school with a group of people, you will only develop the proper preparation and high level of skills if you have the right mindset. It can be tempting to be too laid back or casual, and yes you must enjoy your training, but martial arts is also a serious skill which requires focus and discipline. Nothing is worth doing unless there is one hundred percent effort.

Technical Training

While in your school of martial arts concentrate on what your instructor is saying and doing. Pay complete attention to your training partner and focus on your techniques, performing all of them with effort and physical/mental concentration.

Sparring

There are many different types of sparring – semi, full, striking, grappling, pushing hands and weapons etc. One of the biggest problems when sparring is not only focus but also control of the mind. You should not need to think about what to do, or have thoughts that are irrelevant, that are not productive and may only cloud your mind and hinder your response in combat. Having control of your mind also helps you to be in control of your emotions – for example fear, over confidence and impatience are just a few. If you cannot control these emotions then your opponent will take advantage of them and ultimately defeat you.

Exercise Workouts

Even while exercising you will see students looking around, demonstrating a lack of focus. You must learn to be in the moment because only then will you develop. Looking at your martial arts colleagues will not help – it is wasted energy! Why not channel that energy towards yourself. Think about why are you doing the exercises – to be stronger, faster etc. and challenge yourself to do better in each and every class.

Finally, you must believe in yourself. This belief can be drawn from many sources but ultimately will come from the mind through hard training and meditation.

*he
nowing
re not
onfused,
he
umane
re not
vorried
nd the
rave are
ot afraid*

onfuscius

If you have strong self belief and faith in your abilities you can achieve anything and overcome anyone – victory will be yours.

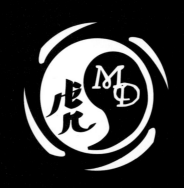

Developing the Mind for Realism

All forms or styles of martial arts work in the right situation. However, when put under real pressure in a dangerous situation most styles would fail. Who is then to blame: the individual or the style?

I think both may be blamed but, as far as style goes, the traditional martial arts are more susceptible to failure than the modern arts. This is because many of their techniques are just too unrealistic and rigid. For example, long stances, forms/katas and complicated movements may take up too much time when a simple head butt or strike to the groin would do. This is not necessarily the case for all traditional styles, but it is very common.

Modern martial arts can be similarly guilty, but their strength is in a more direct and realistic approach to hardcore self-defence for the streets. They have also had the benefit of learning from the more traditional arts and improving on them.

Regardless of the strengths and weaknesses of modern and traditional martial arts it is important to remember that success or failure in a real encounter is more to do with the individual and how they train physically, mentally and spiritually. Cover all the ranges and practice for real situations, which may occur on the street, in a logical, simple and effective way.

Finally, don't get too bogged down with rules when you are training because your opponent is unlikely to abide by them; mix it up and learn to be streetwise – only then will you be prepared for real combat.

'if you are in a confrontation and can walk away then do so. It takes more strength to walk away'

Marc Davis

Fear

Fear is greatly misunderstood.

Many people, within the world of Martial Arts or otherwise, feel consumed by fear. Others will tell you that because of their level of skill or even physical size and strength they no longer have any fear of anyone or any situation.

One of of the most important things in life is to have an understanding of fear because with this comes knowledge, and thus power.

Fear is simply an emotion which we all possess. Try as you may, you can never rid yourself of it. All animals possess fear within them.

Humans and animals often conceal fear to gain an advantage over an opponent as fear itself is seen as a weakness.

As with most things, fear is an emotion and can be trained so that you can control it and prevent it from consuming you and your physical and mental abililty. By controlling fear you can avoid freezing in a threatening situation. Not only that, you can use your control of fear as a very powerful and positive reaction to any situation.

When controlled and directed in the right way, fear can be one of your greatest allies and should be seen as a very positive and powerful force in your arsenal.

Remember, fear is a good thing and above all is used to make you aware of danger, so embrace it rather than fight against it.

'You can never be rid of fear so make it your friend an ally, so that you are in complete control to use it in a positive way '

Marc Davis

What are the Benefits of Sparring?

In martial arts there are so many different areas to practice and so many different styles that all have their own speciality, each one placing greater emphasis on what seems the most important. In this chapter we will look at sparring.

As previously mentioned, there are several forms of sparring. These include chi sau/pushing hands, grappling, weapons and hands and legs (often referred to as freestyle – meaning to use all weapons of the body). Within all these different forms of sparring there is semi-contact, which essentially means controlled fighting, and then there is full-contact, which means you can use full force. Full-contact is governed by rules disallowing strikes to the eyes, throat, groin or joints.

In my opinion semi and full contact sparring are two of the most vital elements of any style of martial arts. No matter how long you have trained for and how many times you practice techniques in a safe and structured way with a willing partner, you will never be fully prepared for full contact sparring or a real fight.

The reasons are endless and obvious – breaking bricks or looking skilled are not a true indication of real skills. The bricks and the punch bag or wooden dummy will not hit you back and will not use angles or tactics to defeat you. Ultimately, they are predictable and lack your most effective weapon in combat – the brain. In freestyle sparring you have a chance to respond to a real person, a skilled individual who will not comply with your wishes and who wants to defeat you.

In conclusion, sparring will help you to develop all the necessary skills and attributes to make your techniques functional and effective both in training and on the streets. It is one of the final and most important levels in order to attain proficiency in body, mind and spirit. Below is a list of the main attributes that you will develop through sparring.

1} Timing 5} Accuracy
2} Rhythm 6} Power
3} Tactics 7} Footwork
4} Speed 8} Control of your emotions
– aggression, fear etc.

'sparring is simply a very physical game where superior tactics of the mind is the most important thing'

Marc Davis

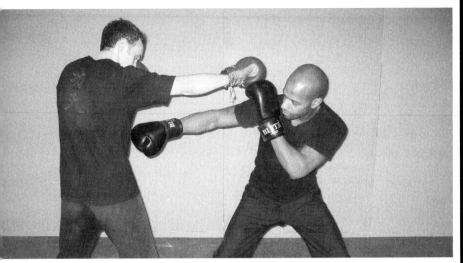

Methods of Sparring

Through the practice of martial arts you learn many different skills such as strikes using all areas of the body; fist, elbows, knees, kicks, shoulder, open hands and the head to name a few. Defence, which involves blocks, parries and evasive movement to avoid an attack. Exercises to strengthen the body and mind, weapons practice and breathing and meditation to help your focus/concentration and to be calm and relaxed in any situation. No matter how many times you practice block and counter with a cooperative partner you will only know your true level of skill through sparring.

There are many different methods of sparring which collectively develop the necessary skills and qualities to be able to defend oneself in free sparring where your partner will not be cooperating with you or in a real life situation. Now lets look at the different types of sparring and their positive and negative points.

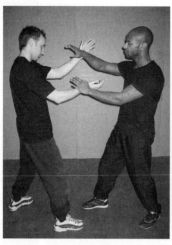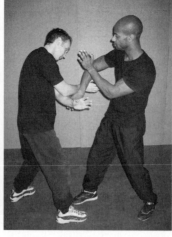

METHOD ONE – Chi sau / pushing hands

This method of sparring emphasises touching of one or both arms and through relaxation sensitivity and sticking with or following your partners movements and energy you spar according to arm pressure, angles, laps of concentration pressure and the intention of your partner.

Positives – develops the correct use of energy, both in attack and defence. Improves timing, speed and close range power.

Negatives – not realistic enough and because you are constantly clinging to each others hands only the close range skills will be developed, but not the medium and long range which means you will not develop the necessary skills to close down your opponent with foot work as well as the entry skills.

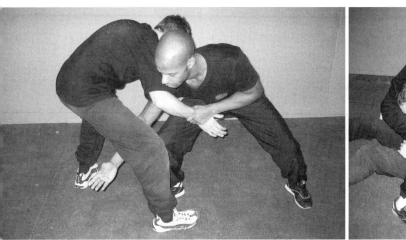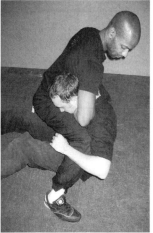

METHOD TWO – Grappling

This form of sparring is practiced from standing, kneeling or the ground position and involves grabbing and clinch work in order to keep your opponent close long enough to throw, choke, lock, pin/restrain or stifle until they are in your control or submit by tapping.

Positives – as many fights can end up on the ground and when the strikes are not available it can be invaluable, it also teaches you how to have good balance and how to unbalance you opponent as well as read and use there energy/pressure against them.

Negatives – Like chi sau it does not go deep enough into footwork and the different ranges. It also does not have striking, which is a major part of any real fight.

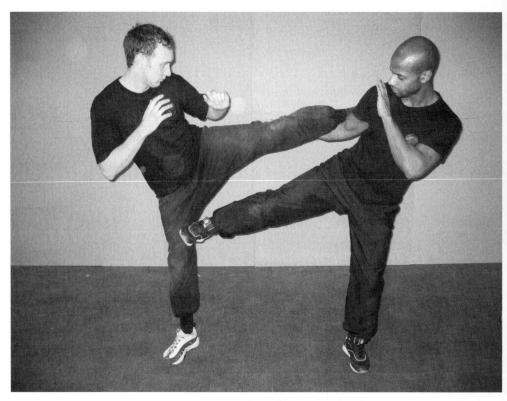

An example of free sparring

METHOD THREE - Hands and legs

In the method of hand and leg strikes often referred to as freestyle you are able to practice the most realistic form of sparring/fighting as you can use punching, open hands, kicks, knees and throws.

Positives – There is the emotional element of over coming your fear of being hit by a full contact strike. The foot work that is required needs to be at the very highest level in order to control the range and close the distance on your opponent to use your strikes.

Ultimately all ranges can be covered in this method of sparring making it the most complete in my opinion.

Negatives – If you do end up on the ground the effectiveness of your strikes may be less powerful, so knowing some grappling techniques could be useful.

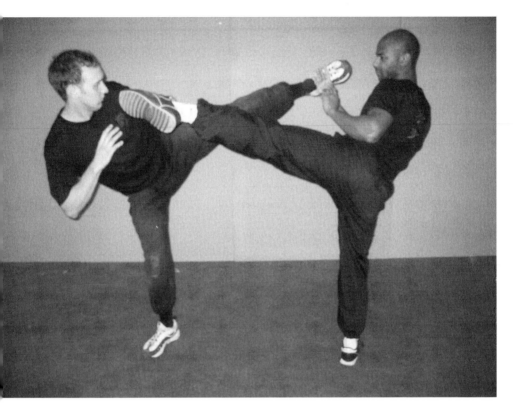

An example of free sparring

Remember regardless of which method you may practice it is best to keep an open mind and be willing to learn all the different ways to spar so you will be more complete.

功夫

Tactics for Sparring

In this chapter we will be discussing the different tactics that can be employed during sparring in a controlled environment - or even a real life situation.

There are endless variables in this subject such as the skill level of the individual and the style they practice. However I will provide an overview of the major elements by discussing some basic and advanced aspects of tactical skills.

First, let's look at tactical methods to employ when making an attack on your opponent; there are nine major areas to attack whether you are at a basic level or advanced. Your ability will determine the nature of your attack..

> *1 High left* – this represents the left and right side of the head/neck such as temple ear or carotid arteries

2 High right

3 Middle left – this represents the left and right side of the body such as the rib cage.

4 Middle right

5 Low left – representing the outer thigh and the knee area.

6 Low right

7 High centre line – represents the eyes, nose, mouth and windpipe.

8 Middle centre line – representing the chest bone, sternum, solar plexus, kidneys and spine.

9 Low centre line – representing the lower abdominal area or the groin.

All of these targets can be attacked in two ways; Method one is direct attack; this means any strike or technique that follows a straight line or path. An example would be a straight jab, a front kick, forward knee or straight finger jab to eyes.

Method two is the indirect attack which utilises circular or curved strikes such as hook punch, inner elbows, turning kicks and so on. Remember - all nine areas apply for both martial arts training and a real fight.

Winning and Losing

This can be a very sensitive area for many people, it is my belief however, that the two are linked and co-exist, just like yin and yang.

You may say that one is positive and the other negative, but ask yourself this, if you do not experience what is negative, for example, losing, how will you truly know and appreciate what is positive.

In order to learn in the martial arts, or indeed life, you must experience losing, and what loss is. You may be at your lowest, but it is from this bottom point that you will truly learn to win and grow. You will then gain a strong foundation, growing steadily upwards and experience winning. You now have experience of both, thus you will make for a stronger opponent. Look at two championship boxers, one is undefeated and is considered one of the best, as good as he may be, his true character and fighting spirit has not been truly tested. Then there is the second boxer who has previously been an undefeated champion.

'defeat is also a state of mind. No one is eve[r] defeated until defeat has been accepted as reality. To me, defeat in anything is merel[y] temporary and its punishment is but an urge fo[r] me to make greater efforts to achieve my goals[.] Defeat simply tells me that something is wron[g] in my doing. It is a path leading to success an[d] truth.' **Bruce Lee**

When he loses, he hits rock bottom, and as history has shown, many boxers or people in any walk of life, and in any job may be so depressed and have such low self-esteem, that they never recover. So if this boxer comes from the depths of despair and wins again, and again, to become a champion once more, then he is strongest. He is the real winner and possesses real fighting spirit and the heart of a champion. But remember – he had to lose to achieve this greatness.

So, just as real life is, full of ups and downs, you must see the negative as a temporary obstacle that you will overcome to become even stronger. Believe in yourself and stay strong in spirit and you will rise to the top again.

'victory is won in mind and spirit even before the fight has begun'

Marc Davi[s]

Pressure Points

Specific areas on the head or body are vulnerable to pressure or being struck. In martial arts these are normally referred to as pressure points.

The result of being hit on a pressure point are varied and ranges from dull or sharp pain to temporary paralysis. In some cases it may even be fatal.

Some pressure points can be found where the nerves are not protected sufficiently, e.g. near the joints or where the skin is thin. However, while this vulnerability is negative in combat, some of these points are also used to treat people who are ill. In Chinese culture it is believed that the body has what are called meridians which run along the nervous system. The principles of yin and yang dictate that if these two forces co-exist in perfect balance and harmony then you will be fit and healthy and a well balanced individual. However if you are sick this means there is an imbalance; too much yin or yang

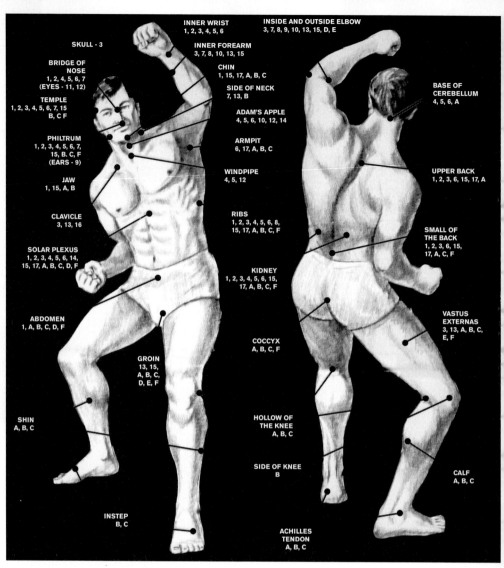

INNER WRIST
1, 2, 3, 4, 5, 6

INSIDE AND OUTSIDE ELBOW
3, 7, 8, 9, 10, 13, 15, D, E

SKULL - 3

INNER FOREARM
3, 7, 8, 10, 13, 15

BRIDGE OF NOSE
1, 2, 4, 5, 6, 7
(EYES - 11, 12)

CHIN
1, 15, 17, A, B, C

BASE OF CEREBELLUM
4, 5, 6, A

TEMPLE
1, 2, 3, 4, 5, 6, 7, 15
B, C F

SIDE OF NECK
7, 13, B

ADAM'S APPLE
4, 5, 6, 10, 12, 14

PHILTRUM
1, 2, 3, 4, 5, 6, 7,
15, B, C, F
(EARS - 9)

ARMPIT
6, 17, A, B, C

UPPER BACK
1, 2, 3, 6, 15, 17, A

JAW
1, 15, A, B

WINDPIPE
4, 5, 12

CLAVICLE
3, 13, 16

RIBS
1, 2, 3, 4, 5, 6, 8,
15, 17, A, B, C, F

SMALL OF THE BACK
1, 2, 3, 6, 15,
17, A, C, F

SOLAR PLEXUS
1, 2, 3, 4, 5, 6, 14,
15, 17, A, B, C, D, F

KIDNEY
1, 2, 3, 4, 5, 6, 15,
17, A, B, C, F

ABDOMEN
1, A, B, C, D, F

VASTUS EXTERNAS
3, 13, A, B, C,
E, F

COCCYX
A, B, C, F

GROIN
13, 15,
A, B, C,
D, E, F

SHIN
A, B, C

HOLLOW OF THE KNEE
A, B, C

INSTEP
B, C

SIDE OF KNEE
B

CALF
A, B, C

ACHILLES TENDON
A, B, C

resulting in a blockage in the meridians. This can be treated by taking Chinese herbal medicine along with what is known as acupressure or acupuncture which involves applying deep pressure by use of fingers, elbows etc or with the use of very small needles on specific points on the body. This pressure stimulates the correct flow of blood and chi and returns the body back to health and a state of balance.

Pressure Points

Joint Locks

Danger of Using Joint Locks and Restraining Techniques

All methods of restraining techniques, be it joint locks, choking or throws are extremely effective but also very dangerous. For example the mind frame of the individuals involved, if the defender is thinking that they will restrain and control but the attacker has other ideas and is simply hell bent on destroying you

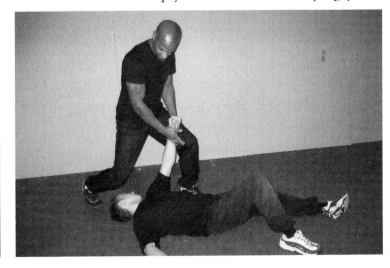

Joint lock
Sifu Marc Demonstrates a painful arm lock

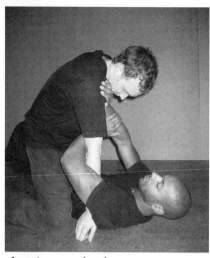

The Figure 4 Elbow Lock

that is not the best strategy to apply. Another point to take in to consideration is if the person that you are trying to restrain is intoxicated, their pain threshold will be much higher than normal thus making the technique harder to apply. You may also find yourself in a situation where you are outnumbered and you cannot afford to be struggling with the first person as there is no time before the others engulf and overpower you. There are many other points to be aware of but I have simply given some of the major ones.

Let me be very clear, this chapter was not written with the intention to belittle the art of joint locking or restraining which involves using leverage against the joints. This will result in causing pain and ultimately breaking of the joint or choking techniques, which can be used to gain control of your opponent as these methods restrict the person's air intake and ultimately the oxygen to the brain, which can be fatal.

With this chapter I am simply trying to highlight the dangers of applying these skills at the wrong time and without the appropriate mind frame and backup techniques thus making the martial artist more aware and in turn able to develop their techniques to a much more effective and efficient level.

'If you do not give your opponent anything to use against you, then what can they do.'

Marc Davis

Deep Breathing – Chi gong

This is the development of your internal power, otherwise known as chi in China, Ki in Japan and prana in India.

The Breath Power, or Power of Breath is our life force found in all living things. By practicing breathing skills we learn to coordinate our internal breathing power with our external movements for example, punching and kicking.

Let us look at some of the methods used to develop this skill/power.

There are many techniques but it is my belief that the root of this power is natural breathing practiced with more depth. Specifically, one breathes from the Dan Tien, the lower stomach, as opposed to the chest.

Chi gung

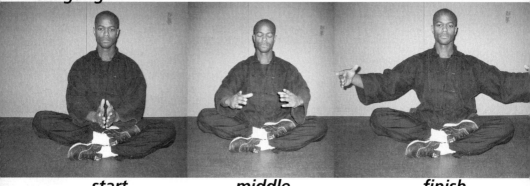

start   middle   finish

Method 1

Sometimes referred to as reverse breathing, this involves relaxing the whole body and breathing in through the nose; as you do so your abdomen (diaphragm) should expand. As you exhale also through the nose your Dan Tien retracts to its natural state.

This method is used for relaxation, calmness, focus, meditation as well as everyday life.

Method 2

This method can be performed in two ways. The first is when you breath through the nose while your muscles are relaxed and exhale through the mouth when muscles are used in striking. Use this method when your movements that require power upon the moment of contact combining external techniques with internal energy.

The other way of performing this method involves breathing in through the nose and out through the mouth slowly as you contract all or specific muscles that you are training to strengthen. You coordinate your skills or body movements with your breathing. These movements are normally performed slowly in order to develop the muscles, tendons and bones.

'victory is won in the mind and spirit even before the fight has began.'

Marc Davis

Meditation

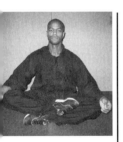

There are many different forms of meditation, such as moving, stationary, using the mind, or even visual meditation. Regardless of which method you choose, the ultimate aim is still the same, to achieve calmness, control and to improve one's concentration and gain awareness between mind, body and spirit.

It is important to note that the mind is the most effective and valuable weapon that we have, everything that we attempt physically must first come from the mind. I like to think of the mind and body as master and servant, to put it another way, if you have a very old computer that once you type in a command there is a long delay before you receive the response, this is down to an old computer that has limited power. If we replace this old computer with a modern computer your command will receive a

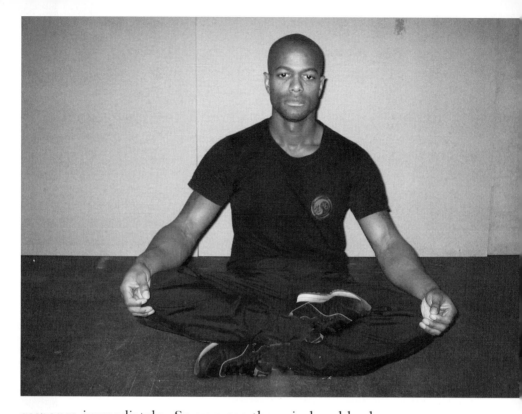

response immediately. So you see the mind and body should be instant. This high degree of response and awareness between mind and body for many martial artists is never fully achieved and their training remains purely physical, as do their skills. This is a novice level, you have achieved only half of the journey compared to the expert who has total control and awareness over mind and body, thus thought and response. As a martial artist and in all areas of your life, the rewards and gains from attaining such a high state of togetherness are endless. For example, you will become a much stronger person as a whole and be able to better control your emotions and overcome your greatest fears.

For the purpose of this book, I will concentrate on three of the most effective methods of meditation that will start you on the road to the journey within.

Method one:

Keep the eyes closed during this method. This is the standing tree posture/method. Simply stand with your feet shoulder width apart, knees slightly bent and your palms placed on your lower abdomen (your Dan Tien point – the storage place for your chi). Rather then let your mind run away and loose focus try to concentrate on one thing of your choice. Inhale and exhale through the nose and try to maintain the position for about fifteen minutes. As time goes on your mind will become stronger, and you will be able to extend this time as you see fit.

Method two:

Youe eyes should be open, but relaxed for this method. You must be sat comfortably with a strong upright posture, again place the hands at the Tan Tien. Visually select something in front of you that is quite small, but that you can clearly see. As you gaze at your chosen object nothing else must enter your mind. Once again breathe evenly through the nose for at least fifteen minutes, building this up as your focus and concentration improves.

Method three:

Your eyes should remain open and focused. This method is called moving meditation. As mentioned before in this book mind, body and spirit must be as one, therefore if you are practicing your physical techniques without mind and spirit, your technique is simply an empty shell. Regardless of what style you do, when practising your strikes, defences or even your forms or katas, be in the moment, a state of total focus and concentration and you will gain the rewards of true technique that comes from the spirit within. However long you choose to train or practice your martial arts, then that is how long you should be focused and in a state of meditation and total awareness. Through dedicated training you will learn to connect with your spirit/Chi and elevate or project your power at will.

'Look within and beyond to see their fears and insecurities.'

Marc Davis

Drills, Forms, Katas and Patterns

In this chapter we will be looking at prearranged techniques which are performed in a specific order.

This method of training varies in name according to the origin of the style, for example in china this method is called forms, in Japan they are called katas and in Indonesia they are known as jurus. Regardless of the name the principles are the same, the sequence of movements is practiced as a way of learning and perfecting the techniques within the style. Once this is learnt the master will then break the forms down and reveal the application of the movements i.e. what they are used for.

The main reason for this chapter is simple; are forms a necessary part of martial arts?

First, let's look at the benefits that can be gained through the practicing of forms. As there are so many movements you of course develop a very good memory. Power, speed and balance are all improved through the constant repetition of the techniques within the forms. One also develops the spirit and improves concentration through performing forms against an imaginary opponent.

I am a strong believer in realistic martial arts and realistic training. This practical approach only leaves room for the essential and absolute minimum; therefore in the MD system of martial arts we have no forms as I believe they are too rigid and set. In a real fight you need to be fluid and totally free to express yourself and, as we are all different, that expression should also be different. The constant repetition of forms can lead to robotic similarities in practicioners.

In MD martial arts we go straight to the application of techniques so that we understand how they are used. This prepares the individual for real combat as the training is constantly done in a live situation and with a real opponent forcing you to adapt to constantly changing circumstances.

'study without thinking and you are blind. Think without study and you are in danger'

Confuscius

Basic Hand/Arm Strikes

Basic Hand Striking Techniques

The different types of hand strikes that are used in Chinese martial arts are very diverse compared to western boxing. For example in western boxing you have many rules and are only allowed to strike your opponent in specific areas with your fist, where as in Chinese kung fu most styles have only a few rules, whereas the MD system has none and you can strike not only with your fist or side of fist, but also the heel, palm, knife edge, elbows, shoulders and even fingers to any part of the opponents face or body.

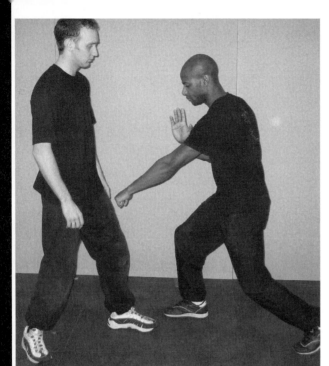

1 – Vertical Punch

This technique is used mainly towards your opponents groin and thigh or if you have thrown them to the floor you can strike to any target.

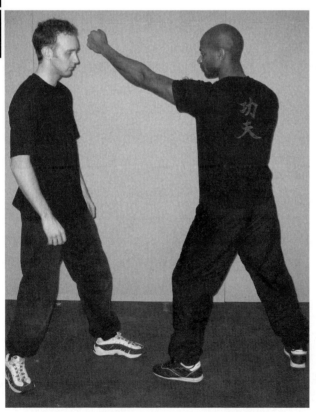

2 – Side Back Fist

When using this technique you strike with the side of the fist towards the opponent's nose, temple or neck. The thing that sets this strike apart from other more conventional strikes is that it can be used from various different types of angles, as it is flexible in direction.

– Reverse
unch

his technique is
pplied by using the
ar hand in a close
nge striking with
e knuckles to the
bs, kidneys, solar
xes and eyes. Make
t just before
mpact for maximum
ower.

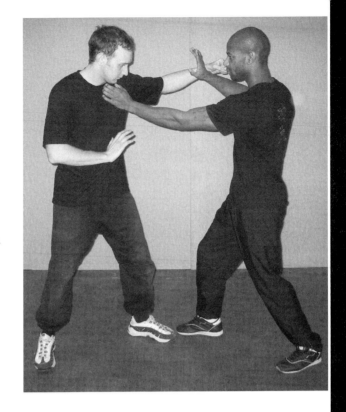

– Vertical Back
st

his strike can be
ed from medium
d close range
ing the back of the
nuckles to strike
e eye or nose,
;ain like the side
ck fist the strike is
so very flexible in
rection and is very
eceptive.

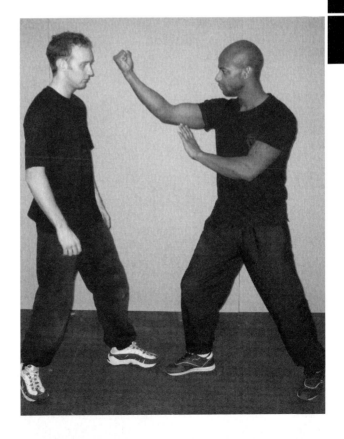

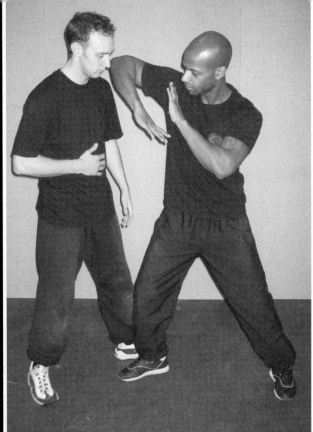

1 – Inner Elbow

This strike starts from a central position and swings inward to its target, which is normally the temple, chin, nose or chest.

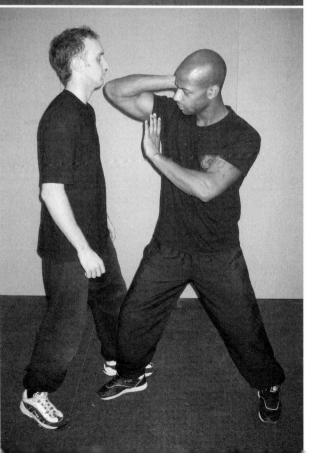

2 – Upward Elbow

Striking in a upward direction towards your opponents chin or nose.

– Vertical Elbow – This techniques follows a downward motion ing the tip of the elbow towards the head, neck, kidney or spine.

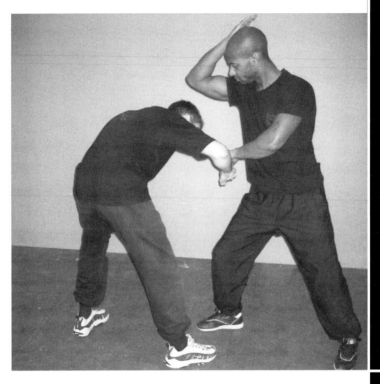

– Backward Elbow – In most cases this strike will be used ainst an attack from the rear. Using a short sharp backward motion ike with the tip of the elbow to the ribs, stomach or head.

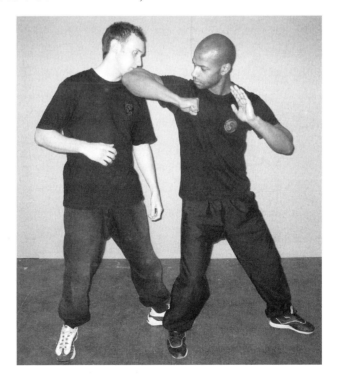

1 – *Palm Down Chop* – This technique utilises the edge of the hand, striking towards the neck, temple, nose and ribs.

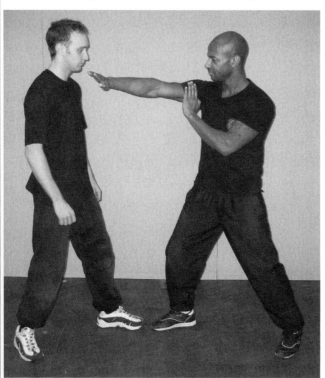

2 – *Reverse Knife Hand* – In general this technique is only used against an attack from the rear. striking to the opponents groin or thigh.

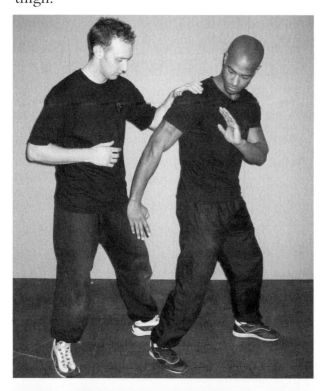

– Heel strike

his technique uses
e heel of the hand
  target the
ponents nose,
mple, chin or
est.

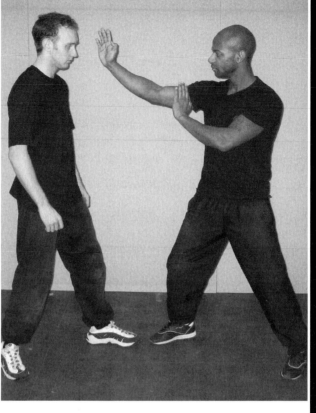

– Palm Up Chop

his technique is the
me as the palm
wn except it can
 used from
fferent angles to
ack the nose,
mple and the neck.

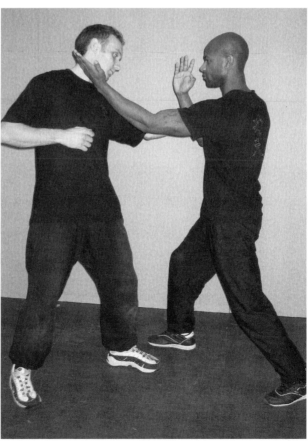

虎

Basic Leg Strikes

This involves using the knee or foot to attack or defend depending on the situation.

Within the martial arts there are four ranges, the knee is for close range strikes and kicks are long-range weapons.

Knee Strikes

 1 Forward
 2 Upward
 3 Cross
 4 Vertical

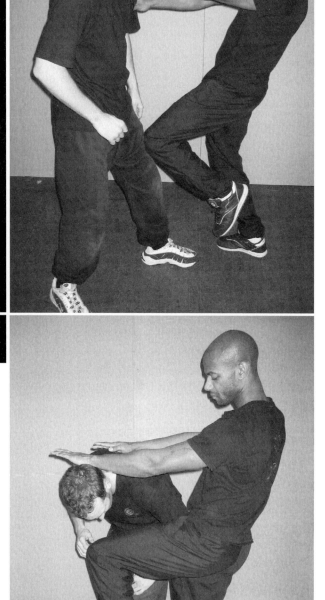

1 – Forward

This is often used to strike the groin, thigh and stomach.

2 – Upward

Target areas are chest and face

– Cross

rget areas are the
ner and the outer
igh

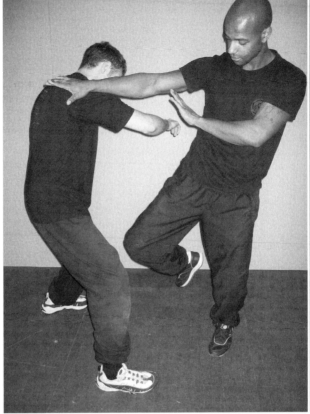

– Vertical

his strike is applied
hen the opponent
 on the ground to
e groin, head and
est.

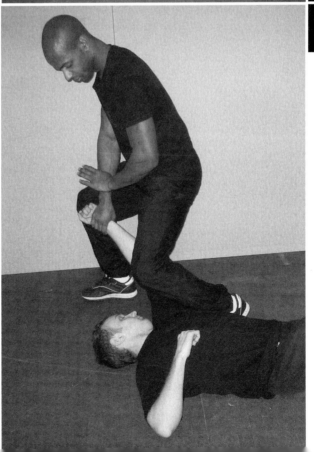

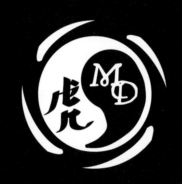

Intermediate Hand Strikes

The difference between basic hand strikes and intermediate or advanced is often to do with the different levels of power that can be generated and the degree of pain inflicted, as well the expected level of difficulty in performing these strikes under pressure.

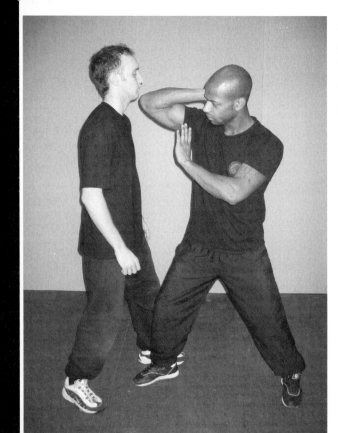

Upward Elbow strike

Targets to aim for would be the chin or nose.

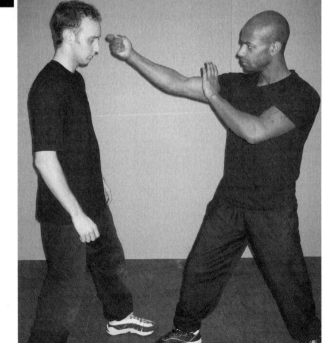

Phoenix Finger

Striking the temple or eye of opponent. this method is mainly used on pressure points or vulnerable areas of the body.

Refer to page 55

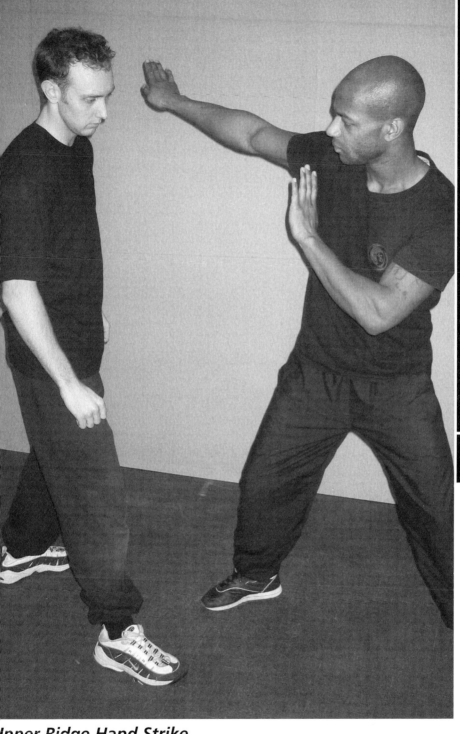

Inner Ridge Hand Strike

Using the edge of the thumb along the heel of the hand to strike the temple or side of neck.

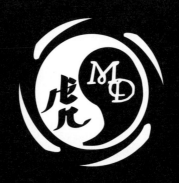

Intermediate Leg Strikes

As mentioned in the previous chapter the level of strikes, in this case kicks, will be the same taking into account the section of the foot that is used and the angle or height that the technique is performed from.

1 – *High Hook Kick* This technique uses the heel of the foot to strike the opponent on the back of the head.

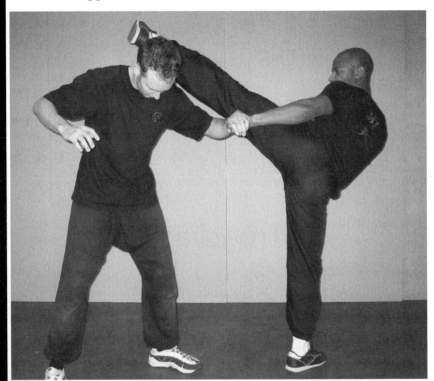

2 – *High Turning Kick* Using the instep of the foot to strike the opponents jaw or temple.

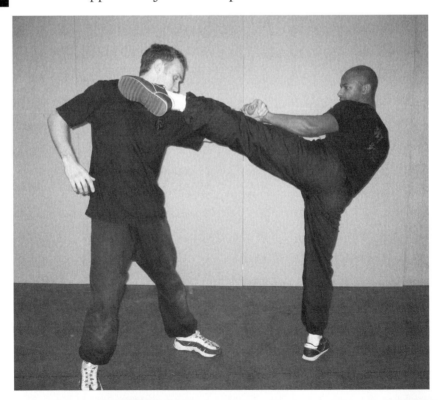

– _Low Side Kick_ Using the heel of foot striking the opponents knee or thigh

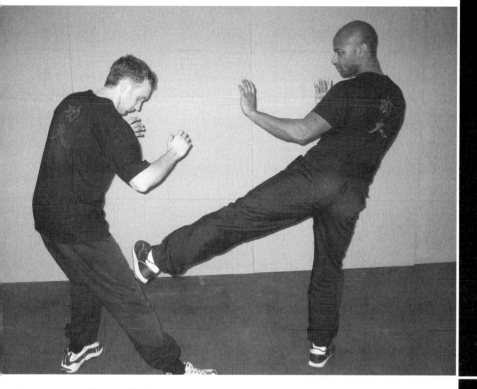

– _Low Turning Kick_ Using the instep striking opponents thigh

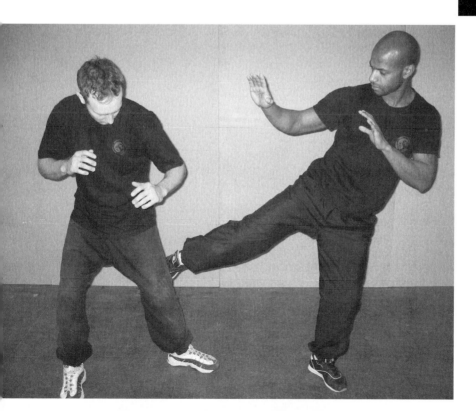

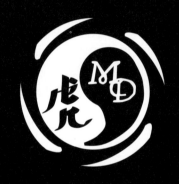

Advanced Hand Strikes

Closed Fist
1 Inner hammer fist
2 Phoenix fist

Elbow Strikes
1 Forward elbow strike
2 Circular elbow

Open Hands
1 Palm hand strike
2 Forward Ridge hand
3 Finger strike

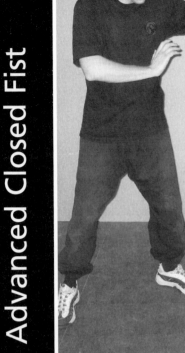

1 – Inner Hammer Fist

This uses the side of the fist in an inward or outward motion to target the temple, nose or jaw.

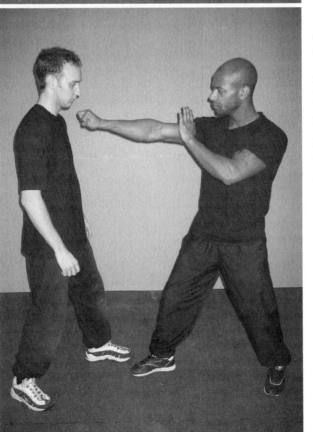

2 – Phoenix Fist

This is one of the most advanced open hand strikes as it requires strong fingers and knuckles to target the eyes, temple, solar plexes and ribs.

– Forward
bow Strike

his is one of the
ost deceptive
bow strikes in the
D system. It is
ed from an
xtremely close
nge, with a short
rward thrust
rected to the chest.

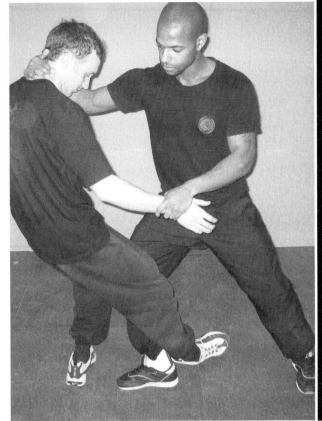

– Circular
bow

he power of this
bow comes from a
rcular downward
otion directed to
e opponents face
r the back of the
ead.

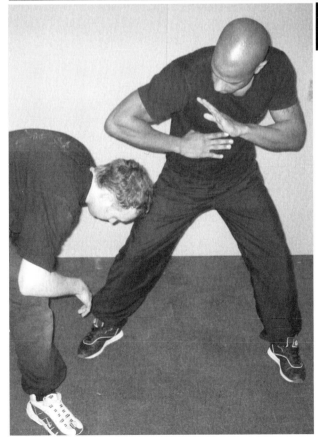

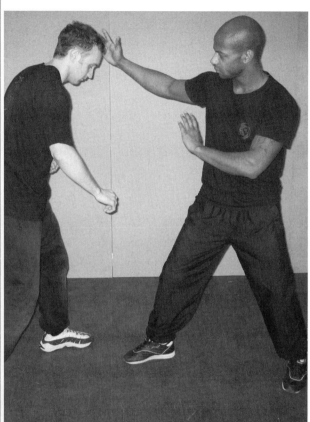

1 – Palm hand strike

This is also one of the most powerful and flexible strikes, as it can be used from almost any angle targeting any part of the body.

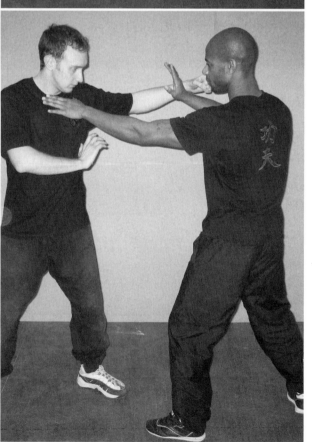

2 – Forward Ridge Hand

This is using the section between index finger and thumb to strike opponents throat. This method is also used in the snake style of Kung Fu.

– Finger strike

his is often
garded as one of
e most advanced
rikes as it uses the
ngers/ fingertips to
rike the opponent.
his requires great
rength in the
ngers. The target
eas are normally
e eyes and throat.

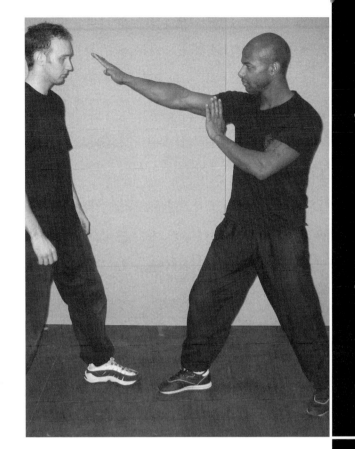

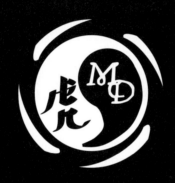

Advanced Leg Strikes

It is important for me to point out that in a real combat situation low line kicking techniques would be the most effective. However, if you are to develop your full potential it is important to posess the skill and technique of advanced level leg strikes. Posessing a very high level of high kicking skills will make your lower line kicks near perfect.

1 Knee- sweep – the emphases is to unbalance and throw your opponent by weakening the inside of his knee.

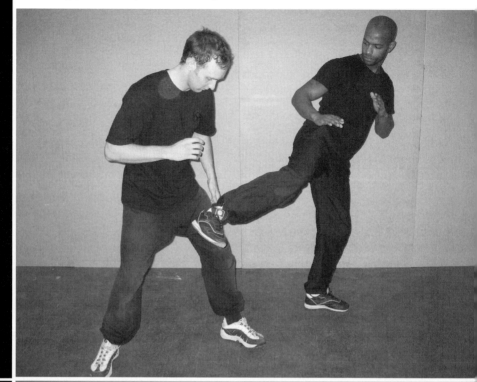

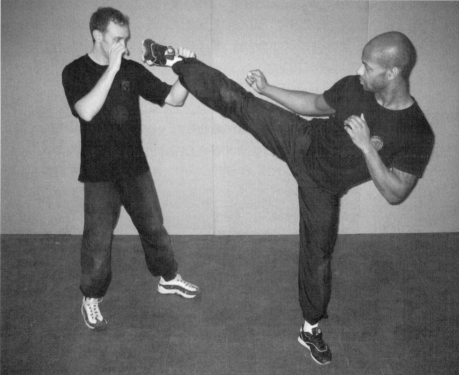

2 High side kick – Using the heel of the foot to strike to opponents chin or nose. This is one of the most direct kicks in martial arts whether used high or low.

Back kick – use the heel of the foot, and strike to groin or knee. This kick is best used against an attack from behind.

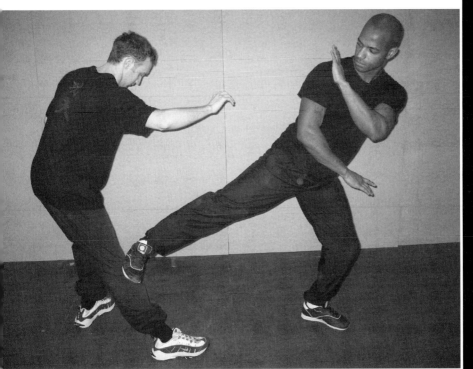

1 Knee- sweep – the emphases is to unbalance and throw your opponent by weakening the back of his knee.

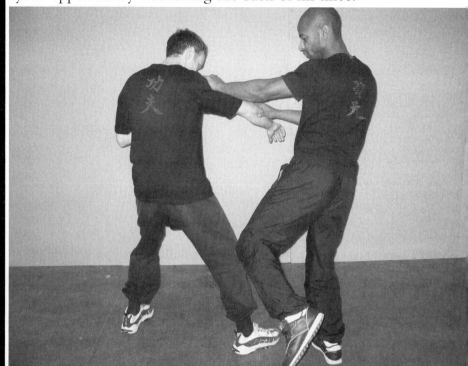

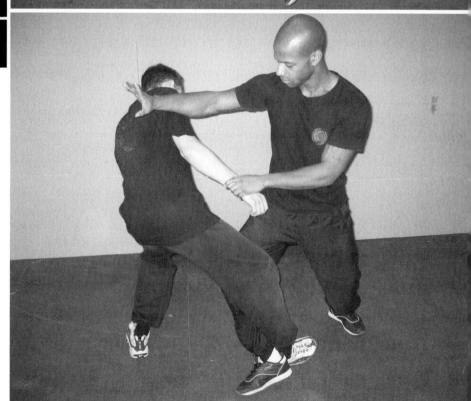

2 Heel hook/trip – use your heel and attack the lower leg of your opponent ending in a leg trip.

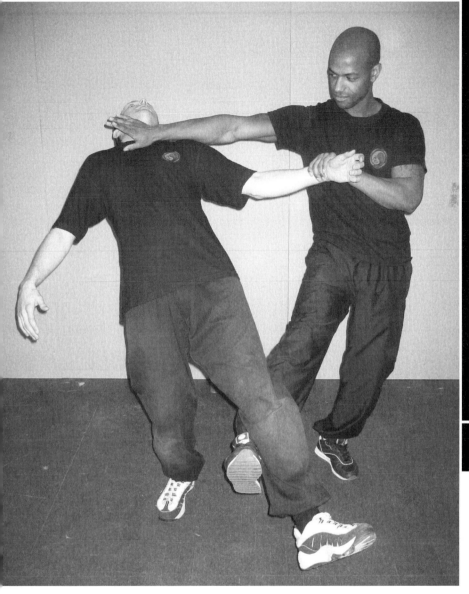

Foot sweep – this technique is to kick your opponent's foot
sing your instep in order to throw them.

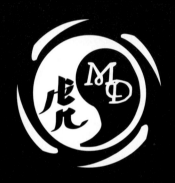

Defence and
Counter

This chapter covers

Defence and counter against knife attacks and also unarmed attacks from behind.

*emember -
'o not
ocus only
n the
nife but
lso on the
erson
olding the
nife as
hey are
1e real
anger*

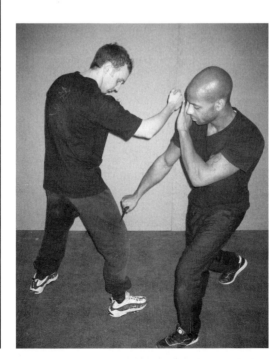

*Evasive
movement*

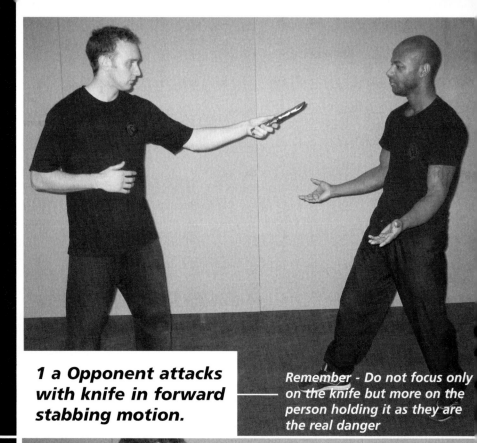

1 a Opponent attacks with knife in forward stabbing motion.

Remember - Do not focus only on the knife but more on the person holding it as they are the real danger

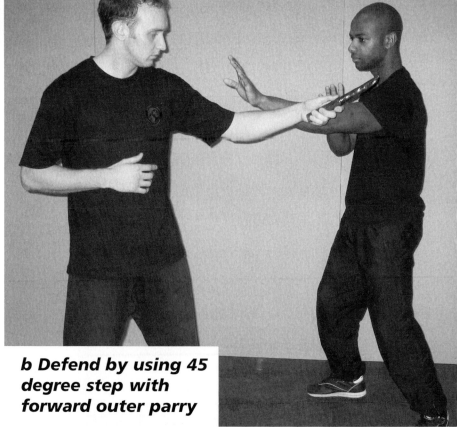

b Defend by using 45 degree step with forward outer parry

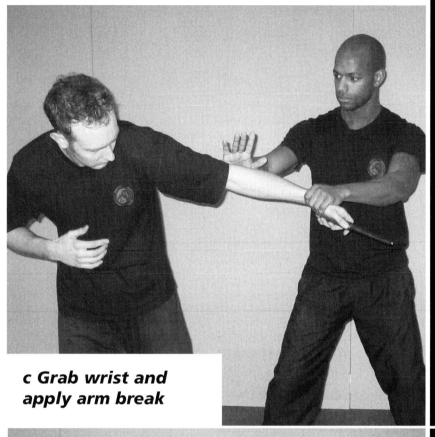

c Grab wrist and apply arm break

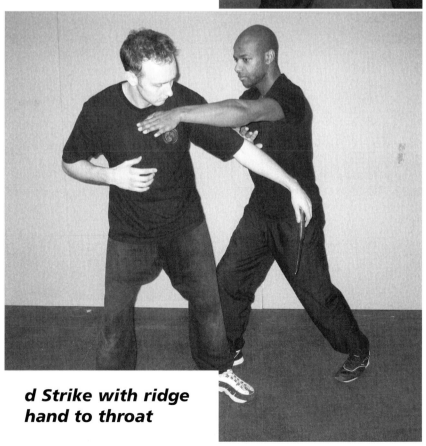

d Strike with ridge hand to throat

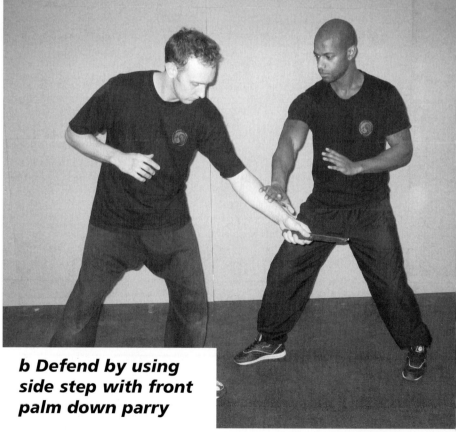

2 a Opponent attacks with knife in forward motion towards stomach.

b Defend by using side step with front palm down parry

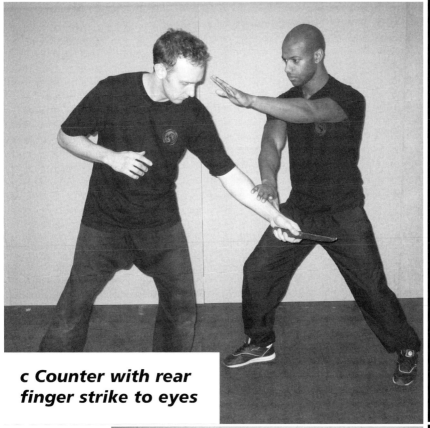

c Counter with rear finger strike to eyes

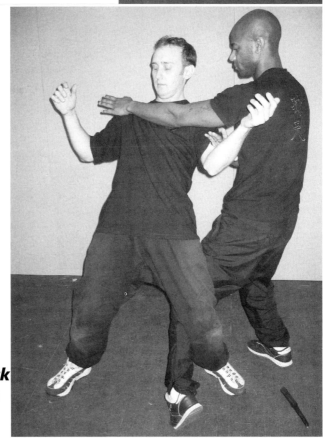

d Throw using rear leg to circle/attack opponents front leg

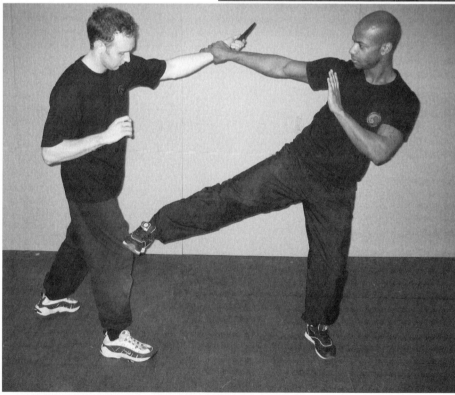

3 a Opponent attacks from the side extending knife as a threat.

b Defend by using inside parry, grab knife hand and apply low side kick to opponents knee

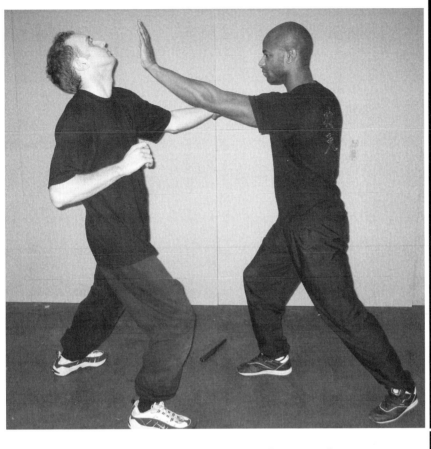

c Finish with rear heel strike to the nose

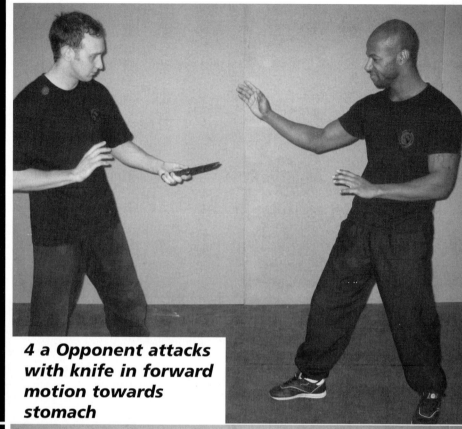

4 a Opponent attacks with knife in forward motion towards stomach

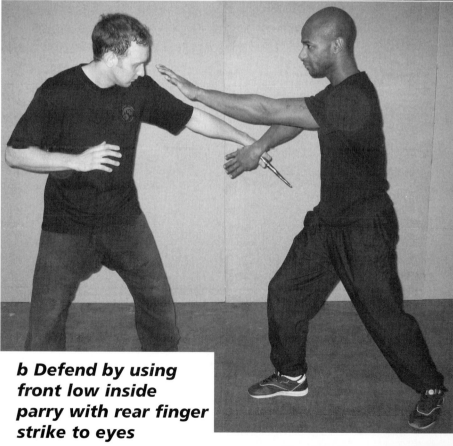

b Defend by using front low inside parry with rear finger strike to eyes

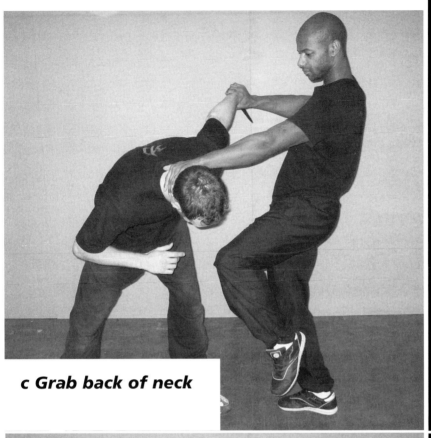

c Grab back of neck

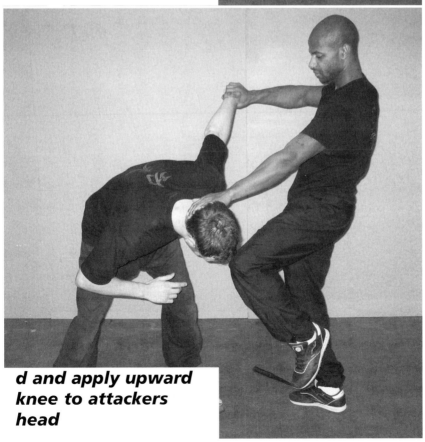

d and apply upward knee to attackers head

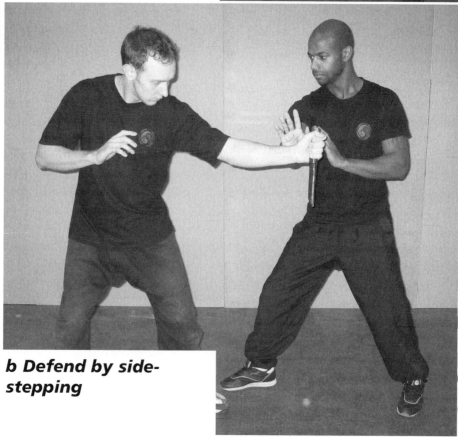

5 a Opponent attacks with knife in a downward motion

b Defend by side-stepping

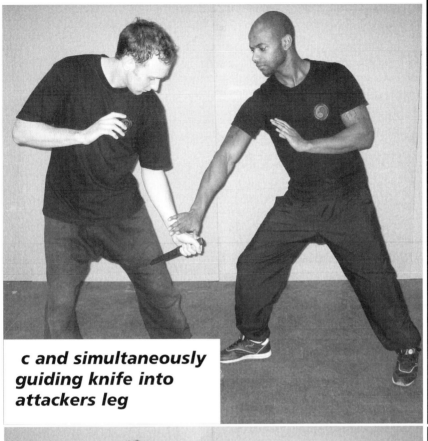

c and simultaneously guiding knife into attackers leg

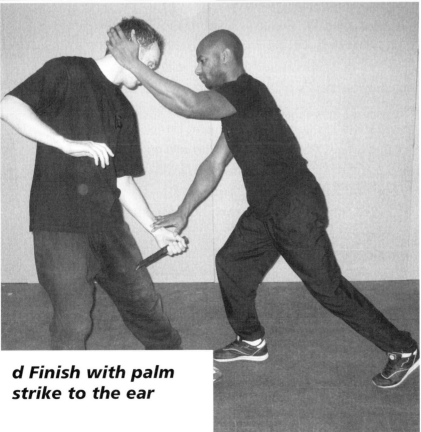

d Finish with palm strike to the ear

Whenever the discussion of knife attacks come up, you often get very complicated and long winded movements. The first thing that should be addressed is if at all possible, run, as the saying goes you will live to fight another day. It is very important to be aware of the value of your life and life itself. So with this in mind, give the attacker/mugger what they want especially if it is only money or jewellery as they are only material things and are not worth your life. If you cannot get away or the attacker does not intend to leave and you have cooperated, you must defend yourself in the most direct and effective way possible. Try to keep your distance because if you can control the range then you can limit the options your attacker has with the knife or any other weapon. Do not focus only on the knife as you can be caught out with a punch or kick, this is a very common mistake. Finally, use anything you can get around your arm to protect it from the knife as you defend yourself, until an opportunity presents itself for you to strike. Or maybe throw something at your attacker to distract them long enough for you to disarm them or escape.

'one of the highest levels of martial arts is avoidance'

Marc Davis

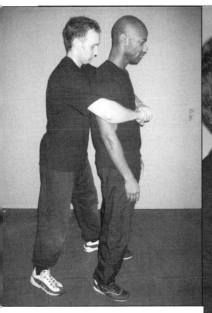

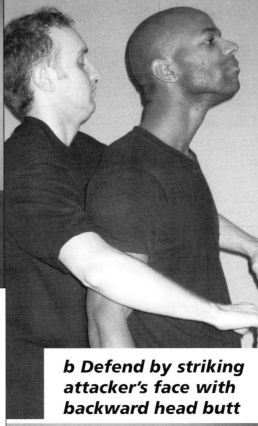

1 a Opponent attacks by grabbing around the arms and body – try to gain immediate sight of your attacker to assess how you are going to respond

b Defend by striking attacker's face with backward head butt

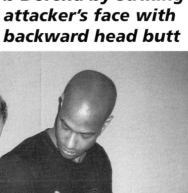

c Follow with a reverse knife hand strike to attacker's groin

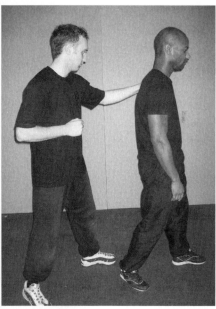

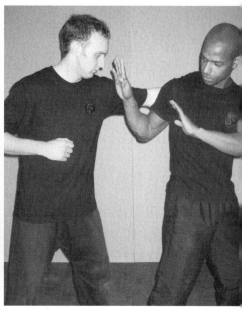

2 a Opponent attempts to grab shoulder

b Defend by turning and using finger strike to eyes

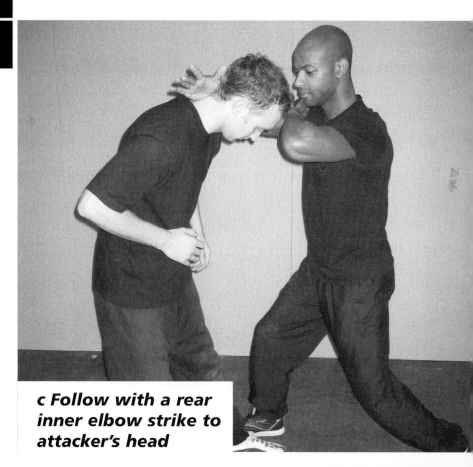

c Follow with a rear inner elbow strike to attacker's head

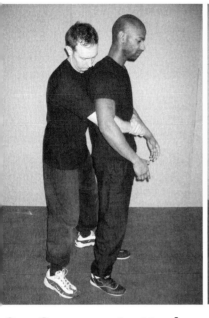 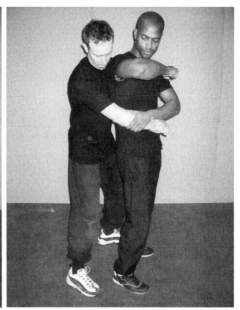

3 a Opponent attacks by grabbing around the body

b Defend by grabbing arm with an elbow strike to the face

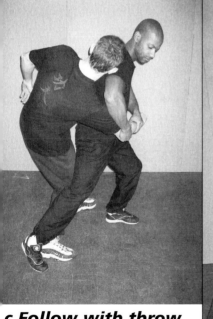 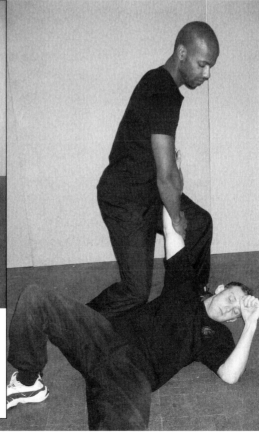

c Follow with throw keeping hold of your opponents arm so you are in complete control

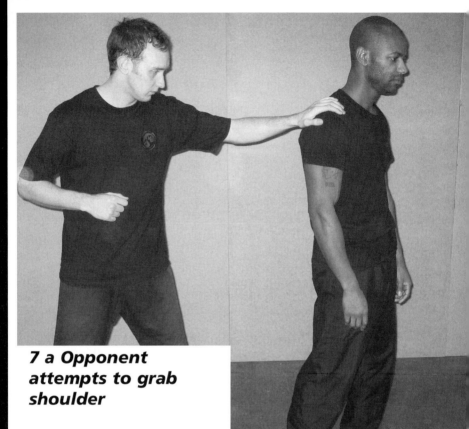

7 a Opponent attempts to grab shoulder

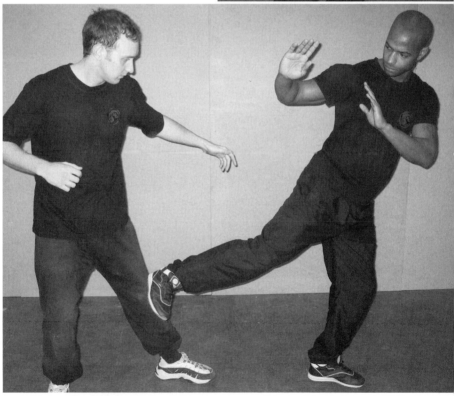

b Defend with low back kick to the knee

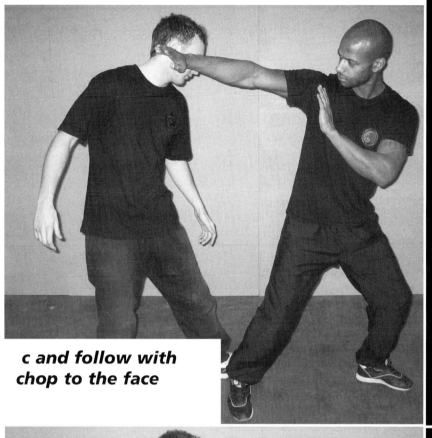

c and follow with chop to the face

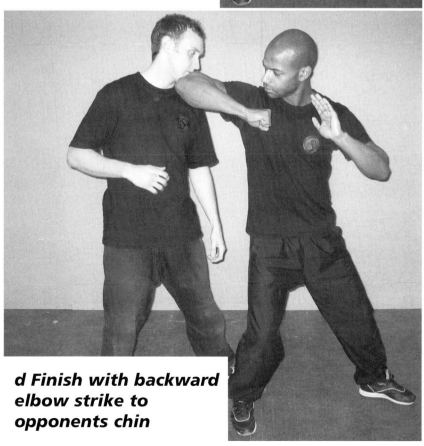

d Finish with backward elbow strike to opponents chin

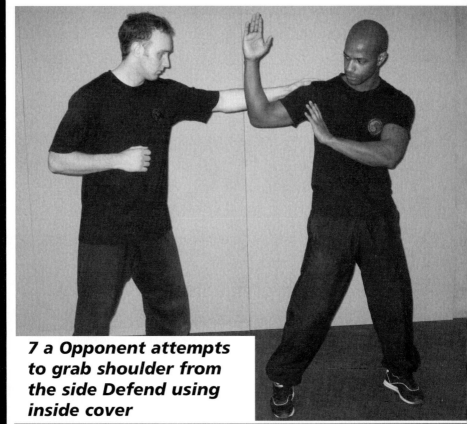

7 a Opponent attempts to grab shoulder from the side Defend using inside cover

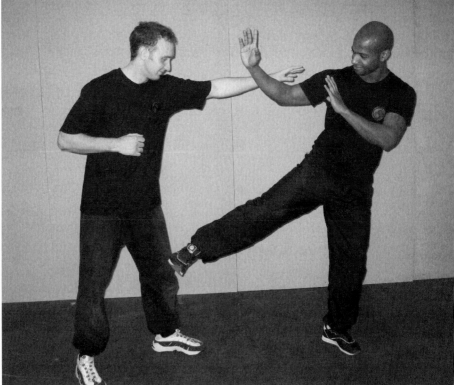

b Strike with low side kick

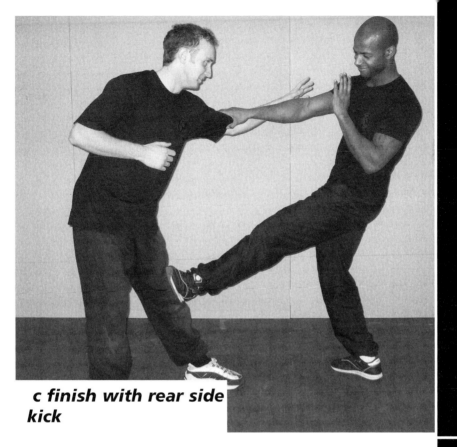

c finish with rear side kick

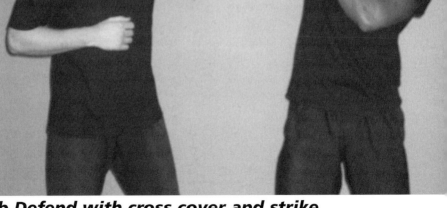

7 a Opponent grabs from the side - try to gain immediate sight of your attacker to assess how you are going to respond

b Defend with cross cover and strike with reverse claw hand

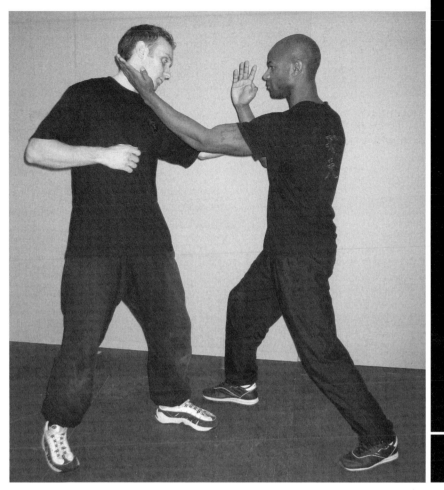

c finish with rear palm up chop while monitoring opponents arm.

Finding a Style that Suits You

When deciding to start practicing a martial art, the first choice you have to make is finding a style that suits you.

There are many things to consider such as the type of person you are, if you are very spiritual, technical and seek the deeper meaning behind things then you will be more drawn to the internal arts for their spirituality, very technical movements and their philosophy.

There is also the physical body and your age to consider. If you are not a particularly physical person or are in your more mature years you may find the softer arts like bua qua, tai chi or aikido more suitable. This is not to say that these styles are not effective or physical enough, but simply that they rely more on technique and using the opponent's strength and force against them. It is worth noting that the softer internal arts are held in the very highest regard and are considered by many martial artists as attaining the highest level of power sophistication and effectiveness.

A younger person who enjoys the physical side of things and prefers a simple and direct approach may be drawn to a style like hsing I, pak mei, Thai boxing or shotokan karate.

It is important to note that all styles of martial arts are technical in their own way. However, some rely on physical strength to a much greater degree, while others place greater emphasis on mind, accuracy, evasive angles and non-resistance.

In conclusion, it is important to consider all things about yourself and what you are looking for. Age, weight, height, strength, character, mental and physical attitude as well as what you want and expect out of your style and training may all affect your decision. All styles have something to offer and regardless of which style you choose always keep an open mind and respect all forms of martial arts. Once you have a very strong foundation and understand your chosen style I would advise you to explore other styles and methods in order to make you a more knowledgeable and complete martial artist.

'expression of art is ultimately the expression of self

Marc Davis

Finding a Good Teacher

As soon as you begin your journey within the martial arts, you will have one of the most important decisions to make – you must find a good teacher.

Finding teachers is not hard, but a very good or exceptional one can be harder to track down. It may be a process of trial and error as you learn more about martial arts and witness teachers of different levels and calibre.

The following are just a few guidelines to assist you:

A good teacher should make you feel relaxed and that you can trust and believe in them

They should not be arrogant but confident and able to perform physically, mentally and spiritually to a very high standard.

The teacher should show a level of control, even when sparring with their best student.

Obtain a history of their training background and references.

Don't judge a teacher by how many black belts they have, as these can be bought in shops. Their skill may also vary depending on the level of the person who issued this teacher with their belts or certificates.

Observe the skill level of the teachers students and there behaviour. This is often a good indication of the teacher's skill, both as a practitioner and a teacher remember not all good martial artists make good teachers.

Finally, there is class etiquette; is there a high level of discipline and respect?

Do you feel safe in the surroundings and would you fit in with the specific school and teacher?

'anyone can follow but few can lead, remember even when you lead to be willing to learn'

Marc Davis

Gradings

This can be a touchy subject for many so I will keep it simple. If you gain your black belt through hard work blood sweat and tears, then that achievement really means something and I would fully support you as long as you work for it.

The flipside to this is that some teachers may give belts away every few months. It has become too simple and too commercial to do this and is a way for instructors to keep their students. In this context the belts or grades will mean nothing. With this type of structure it would take on average 2- 3 years to become a black belt. As Bruce Lee once said, belts are only good for holding up your trousers.

It is important to realise that when you leave your martial arts club and take your belt off it does not change the level you are at. The most important thing is the person and ultimately the developments that they make physically, mentally and spiritually.

I cannot stress enough that there are no shortcuts towards the goal of becoming an expert in the martial arts so don't fool yourself. However, with the right teacher, discipline, dedication, sacrifice and a lot of hard work over a period of many years you can achieve your goal. Exactly how long it takes depends on the teacher and the style as some are more difficult than others and contain a lot more in their syllabus. Finally there is the individual, and as we are all different and learn and develop at different levels how long it takes will be different for each person.

The intention of this chapter is simply to make the reader aware that training within the martial arts with the sole intention of gaining belts as quickly as possible is a road to nowhere. Its like working in a job that you don't like – it will be short lived and you will not gain any real satisfaction or like the feeling that you have been given something you did not earn or deserve. To achieve something that you know you really earned and that nobody can ever take away from you is one of the greatest feelings in the world.

No-one will ever be able to take that sense of achievement away from you.

'he who knows when he has got enough is rich'

Lao Tze

Muscle Development Exercises and Workouts

Physical fitness through martial arts training and exercise is very important. This especially important in MD Martial Arts due to the individual nature. It obviously makes sense that the better the condition of the the martial artist, the better they can perform all their skills.

There are many different types of exercises to develop the muscles of the body but it is not just strength you need to build.

Muscle tone
Power
Speed
Muscle endurance
cardio – heart and lungs
Flexibility

These are the main areas of exercise to be concerned

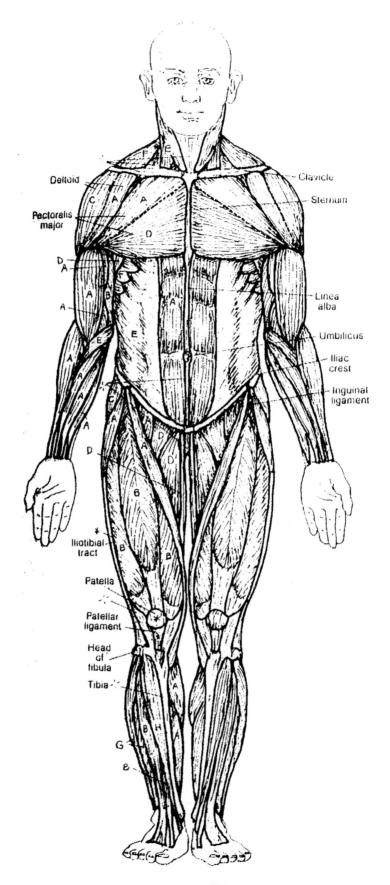

Deltoid

Pectoralis
major

Clavicle

Sternum

Linea
alba

Umbilicus

Iliac
crest

Inguinal
ligament

Iliotibial
tract

Patella

Patellar
ligament

Head
of
fibula

Tibia

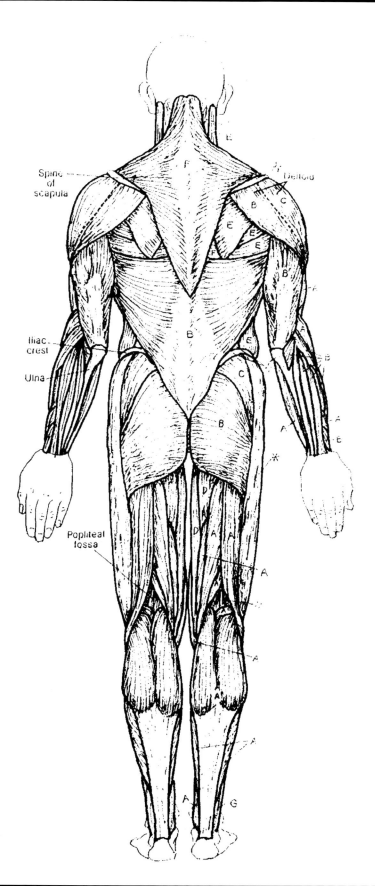

Spine
of
scapula

Deltoid

Iliac
crest

Ulna

Popliteal
fossa

with while training to be a martial artist. it is important to set yourself goals so rather than being strict with number of reps and sets start with something that you can manage and gradually increase the reps and sets as you get stronger month by month until you achieve your maximum goals.

Muscle Tone/Muscle Development

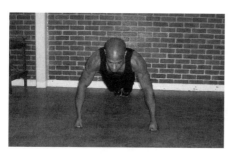 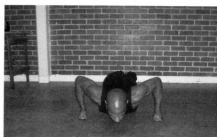

Upper Body

Exercise 1

Chest muscle (Pecs) – Wide Press Ups, 3 sets of 10-20 reps

Exercise 2

2 Person exercise where your partner provides resistance while you try and bring your forearms together. Similar to a Pec Deck or bench press.

Biceps – upper arm muscle

Exercise 1

Isometric – muscle against muscle. Hold one arm at 90 degrees and place other hand on top of forearm as you push up.

Exercise 2

2 person drill. Hold both arms out in front of you at 90 degrees and have your partner apply resistance downward while you curl arm upwards.

Triceps – Back of upper arm

Exercise 1

Place your arm at 90 degrees and place other hand under forearm and apply resistance while pushing down.

Exercise 2

Tricep Dips

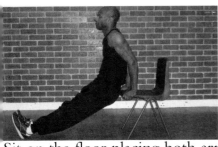
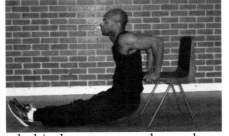

Sit on the floor placing both arms behind you on an elevated surface. Push yourself up and back down slowly. Exercising the triceps can also be done with dumbells in a standing or sitting position and raising and lowering the dumbell behind the head.

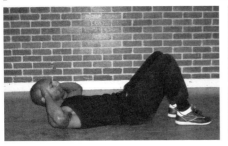
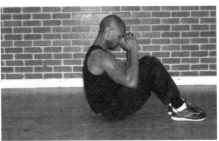

Mid Body

Sit-Ups – abdominal muscles, 3 sets of 20 reps

Exercise 1

Lie on back, knees bent and feet on floor. Using your abdominal muscles raise yourself upwards breathing out and breath in as you lower yourself slowly back down.

Exercise 2

Pelvis Tilts – for lower abdominal muscles

Lie on your back with your legs crossed and at 90 degrees. Place hands palm down on the floor and push your legs upwards using your hips (without rocking) breathing in as you do so and out as you return slowly to the starting position.

Exercise 3

Twisting Sit–Ups – for the oblique muscles (love handles).

Lie on your back with one leg's ankle crossing the other at the knee. Place your hands on your temples and as you raise yourself upwards using your obliques, twist towards knee breathing out. slowly return to starting position breathing in.

Exercise 4

Side Sit-Ups – also for Obliques.

Lie on your side. Knees bent together with hands on your temple. Using your abdominal muscles raise yourself up breathing out and slowly return to starting position breathing in.

Lower Body
Exercise 1

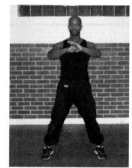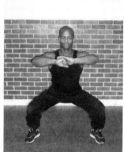

3 sets of 25 reps

Quads/thighs.

Stand with your legs shoulder width apart with knees pointing out slightly as you squat up and down keeping a perfectly straight back.

Exercise 1

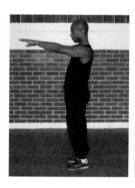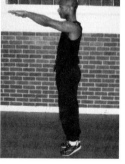

Calf Raises

Stand perfectly upright with feet together. Elevate your body by rolling up onto the balls of your feet and onto your toes and down again. Do not let your heels touch the floor.

Cardio Development Exercises and Workouts

Cardio is aerobic fitness which is designed to increase your heart and lung capacity.

Exercise 1

Jump Jacks/Star Jumps

The starting position is with your feet together and hands by your side. Proceed to jump bringing your arms and legs up and out. Remember to breathe out for jumping and inhale when returning to starting position.

Exercise 2

Knee Jumps

Stand with your feet shoulder width apart with your arms by your side. Jump up into the air and bring your knees up towards your chest using your arms for momentum. Remember to breathe out for jumping and inhale as you return to starting position.

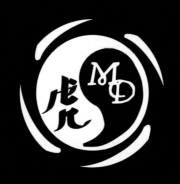

Nutrition
by Dr Amy Davis

Diet is an important part of training and despite there being a great variety of foods available for modern day athletes, most still have the same misconceptions about what foods they should and shouldn't eat and how this will affect their performance. The most common of these misconceptions is that there are magical food products that will enable you to train harder, increase your speed and improve at a faster rate. Unfortunately, there are no such food types. An athlete, just like anyone else, must eat a healthy well-balanced diet.

A well-balanced diet provides all the energy, vitamins, minerals and other nutrients essential to all human life. Food supplies the body with energy; how much energy, or food, a person needs depends on how much energy they use each day. The average man will need around 2550 Kcal per day, whereas the average woman needs only 1950 Kcal per day. When a person is exercising regularly the amount of food, or energy, they need will increase in response to the extra demands placed upon the body.

A well balanced diet should consist of 50% carbohydrate (bread, pasta, rice, potatoes), 35% fat (most foods contain fat) and 15% protein (meat, fish, cheese, nuts) for the average man or woman, along with five portions of fruit or vegetables each day. Try to vary what you eat, this way you can ensure that you are supplying the body with all the vitamins and minerals it needs.

For an athlete who is training regularly their food intake °may be tweaked slightly to cope with the individual exercise regime. For example, if the aim of your training is to improve your stamina, and you are doing endurance training, eating slightly more carbohydrate and protein and slightly less fat may be beneficial. It is a common myth that eating lots of protein helps to improve strength – this is why you will see bodybuilders drinking protein shakes. In actual fact an athlete undertaking heavy strength exercises only needs slightly more protein that the general population, and by eating proportionately more protein than other food types you may actually by causing your body harm.

Having said all of the above is important to note that individual factors also contribute to maintaining a well balanced diet. Each person requires a different amount of food, based on his or her basal metabolic rate. The basal metabolic rate is the minimum amount of energy our bodies need each day to sustain life. It varies between individuals, between the sexes, with exercise and with age. Therefore, a diet should be individual to that person and their needs. This is why fad diets are useless as they are generalised and not specific to the individual.

The sensible way to create a diet for yourself is pay attention to your body and what it needs. If you are gaining weight (and you don't want to) then you are eating too much, if you are losing weight (and you don't want to) then you are not eating enough. You should eat only when you are hungry and, although you should enjoy your food, try not to get into the habit of eating for pleasure as you will no doubt eat too much, and the foods you will enjoy the most will probably not make up a balanced diet.

During exercise the body will utilise different food types preferentially as they are broken down to form energy in different ways. Carbohydrate and fat make up the majority of fuel for the body. An athlete eating a well balanced diet will use relatively little protein as fuel during exercise. Carbohydrate is a much more efficient fuel for the body to use during exercise. Whether or not it is used largely depends on it's availability. There are two different forms of carbohydrate, simple and complex. Simple carbohydrates are found in foods such as white bread, white rice, and chocolate; these foods are broken down and used very quickly to supply energy to the body providing what is known as a 'sugar rush'. Complex carbohydrates, on the other hand, can be found in brown bread, and brown rice. They are broken down much slower and can therefore provide the body with energy for a longer period of time. This will affect the use of fat for energy, in that with simple carbohydrates more fat will need to be used for energy than is the case with complex carbohydrates. This may affect your diet if you are exercising in an attempt to change your body shape.

Fluids are an important part of a well balanced diet, and are particularly important in exercise. As you sweat you are constantly losing water and electrolytes. Small amounts of fluid are also lost when we exhale. This loss is a potential problem as dehydration can reduce your capacity to exercise effectively. An athlete may lose between 1 and 3 litres of fluid when training hard which will need to be replaced. It is important to begin each training session fully hydrated. Trying to adapt to dehydration, and deliberately restricting fluids, will not only reduce the effectiveness of the training session, but may also be dangerous as the risk of heat exhaustion and life-threatening heat-stroke will be greatly increased. This is one instance where just because it feels harder to train, and you are really pushing yourself, it does not mean that it will help you to improve. It is therefore important that you understand the symptoms of dehydration so that it can be avoided. These include, tiredness, headaches and dark coloured urine.

It is important that you find a drink that you enjoy (non-alcoholic!) as this will encourage you to drink more and prevent dehydration. Sports drinks available in shops are ideal for the athlete who is training hard. As we sweat we not only lose water, but also different electrolytes that are necessary for the body to perform at its optimum. Electrolytes are contained in these sport drinks, and so therefore they will also be replaced when drinking them. However it is important to note that many of these drinks also contain sugar, which will provide the body with energy and this must be take into account when thinking about diet, as too much energy intake may lead to an undesirable increase in weight.

Drinking before and during exercise is important to prevent dehydration. Drinking after exercise is important to replace fluid and electrolyte stores in the body and aid recovery, particularly of the muscles. It is also important to replace energy stores after exercise, and the quicker the better. This can be done easily by either eating around 50-100 grams of carbohydrate, for example a banana, or by drinking something containing carbohydrate, for example sports drinks. It is important to replace the electrolytes as well as the fluids, as water alone will not be absorbed into the body effectively and a large proportion of it will be lost into the urine. Try not to drink alcoholic drinks or caffeine based drinks such as tea and coffee as they will also promote loss of fluid into the urine and prevent adequate rehydration. Fizzy drinks will lead to a feeling of stomach fullness, and bloating This will decrease the quantity of fluids you drink, and should therefore be avoided.

The message to take from this is to simply be sensible about what you eat and drink. Try to eat a well-balanced diet with a wide variety of food. Listen to your body, eat when you are hungry and drink when you are thirsty. Make sure that you prepare your body for exercise to prevent dehydration and optimise your training. And most importantly of all, have fun with it and enjoy yourself.

How Long does it take to be able to Defend Yourself?

In many ways this is an impossible question to answer as each person is different and therefore learns and develops in different ways and at different speeds.

The chosen style is also key to the speed of progress as some styles are quite easy to learn while others are more difficult. Another factor is the quality of the teacher and their ability to pass on their knowledge to their students.

As a general guideline, within one year you should notice a definite improvement in awareness, speed, power, accuracy and timing. After this period you will still be at quite a basic level but even at this basic level you should be able to strike with your fist, elbows and knees with a good degree of power. Your effectiveness will still depend on the calibre of opponent and the situation, but you should at least have the necessary tools to stop an attacker. Most importantly, you now have a much greater chance of defending yourself than you would have had twelve months earlier.

I would like to end this chapter by emphasising that you should never put a time limit on the development of your skills; the practice of martial arts requires great discipline and patience. It is a life long journey of growth and perfection of your skills and of yourself. Remember – anyone can win or lose a fight – the purpose of martial arts is to avoid conflict. As your confidence grows and you learn how to fight, you will realise you have nothing to prove and thus be able to walk away from potential trouble. This requires greater strength – the best fighters never fight and the best form of self-defence is not to be there in the first place.

'you will achieve clarity of thought when you posses a clear and peaceful mind'

Marc Davi.

How Long does it take to become Blackbelt/ proficient?

In the last chapter we discussed how long it should take for someone in the martial arts to be able to defend themselves. This naturally leads to another commonly asked question: how long will it take to achieve a black belt? This is the wrong way to look at your training, you should think of the effort you need to put in rather than the time it will take – this will give you a greater sense of achievement and contentment when you eventually achieve a blackbelt.

However, instead of putting in the hard work many people are drawn to shortcuts like grading every few months and the promise of a black belt within two years. This is a very dangerous approach and any self-respecting martial arts teacher would never promote these ideas. To follow this type of structure will ultimately lead to very low quality students and a big wake up call once you branch out and begin to see other schools' students and teachers who have put in the real hard work – blood, sweat and tears over a period of many years.

Being able to demonstrate the required skills physically, mentally and spiritually is the only way to achieve a black belt. If you can do display these qualities you will have earned it and no-one will ever be able to take that away from you. The time it takes to gain a black belt or reach an expert level is different for each of us as we are all different. It also depends on the skill of the teacher and what style you study, as some are very easy to learn and others very difficult. The Chinese have a saying: ten years study within the martial arts will give you some good basics!

Finally, I would like to discuss a very misunderstood point; many people both within and outside of the martial arts think that when you achieve your black belt there is nothing more to learn and that that is the end of your training. Nothing could be further from the truth. In my opinion gaining a black belt simply means you should possess a degree of proficiency physically and mentally. You are now at an open door, which leads to many new discoveries, a deeper understanding of martial arts as well as its techniques, spiritual growth and understanding. Ultimately, one strives for complete knowledge and understanding of oneself and thus others and seeks to perfect the finer points of external and internal techniques which require minimum effort but yield maximum results. The journey of martial arts is not about how long it takes to get a belt, be it two, three or even ten years but is rather a life long pursuit of excellence, growth, discovery and mastery of oneself. Very few people are concerned with or willing to continue their training within the martial arts after a black belt but I can assure you that the rewards are truly great. After twenty-three years of martial arts training I am still walking this path of knowledge.

I leave you with these few words – no-one knows it all, stay humble and always be willing to learn more.

o-one
nows it all,
ay humble
nd always
e willing to
arn more'

Marc Davis

Great Martial Artists

Founders of Popular Martial Art Styles

 Bruce Lee – founder of jeet kune do (meaning intercepting fist)

His art was developed through his study of many different forms of martial arts and his experiences in life. It is an individual process and not a style.

 Kou tze – developed monkey style kung fu

This style focuses on low stances/postures and deceptive techniques and evasive movements.

 Wado ryu karate was developed by hironori ohtsuka

Unlike many styles of karate – wado ryu focuses gretalty on body shifting in order to avoid force against force and turning it's blocking techniques quickly into strikes.

Tang soo do is a Korean martial art that was developed by hwang kee

This style is both hard and soft, emphasizing strikes, throws, locks and the use of weapons

Shukukai karate was founded by chojiro tani

The emphasis is on speed and mobility.

Shotokan karate was developed by gichin funakoshi

This style is known for it's powerful blocks and striking techniques.

Goju ryu karate was founded by chojun miyagi

This style means hard and soft. It has a strong influence of Chinese kung fu.

Mantis kung fu was founded by wong long

Developed in southern china, it focuses strongly on grabbing techniques and clawing as well as punching and kicking skills.

Wing chun was developed by ng mui

This is a southern style of kung fu that uses simultaneous defence and counter techniques. It focuses on close range fighting and all kicks are below the waist.

Aikido was developed by morihei ueshiba

This is a very evasive style that yields to the opponents force and utilises throws, locks and pinning techniques- with great focus on Ki, power/energy.

Chen style tai chi founded by chen wong ting

Tai chi chuan means grand ultimate fist. Slow graceful movements, utilising the whole body and emphasising the development of chi energy. (tai chi is moving meditation)

Judo was developed by jigoro kano

Rather than striking the opponent, judo techniques focus on throws and holds. Using the opponents strength against them in order to control them.

Kempo karate was introduced by james m mitose.

Emphasis on the attacking of pressure points. Techniques used are rapid strikes with hand or foot, throws, locks and take-downs.

Boxers

Boxing Champions

In the world of martial arts boxing is held in very high regards, especially with the styles that emphasise full contact training. Boxers are respected because it is a full contact skill with a scientific approach to combat. The 'sweet science' of boxing as it is called has produced some of the greatest fighters and boxing champions in history. The following list is a tribute to some of these great warriors.

Heavyweight

Muhammed Ali
Fights: 61
Wins: 56
Losses: 5
Draws: 0

Joe Lewis

Fights: 67

Wins: 64

Losses: 3

Draws: 0

Mike Tyson

Fights: 47

Wins: 45

Losses: 2

Draws: 0

Joe Frazer

Fights: 37

Wins: 32

Losses: 4

Draws: 1

Jack Dempsey

Fights: 81

Wins: 66

Losses: 6

Draws: 9

Jersey Joe Walcott

Fights: 72

Wins: 53

Losses: 18

Draws: 1

Floyd Patterson

Fights: 64

Wins: 55

Losses: 8

Draws: 1

Jack Johnson

Fights: 108

Wins: 86

Losses: 10

Draws: 11

No contest: 1

Gene Tunney

Fights: 83

Wins: 62

Losses: 1

Draws: 0

No decisions: 19

Rocky Marciano
Fights: 49
Wins: 49

Middleweight

Sugar Ray Robinson
Fights: 202
Wins: 175
Losses: 19
Draws: 6
No contest: 2

Sugar Ray Leonard
Fights: 39
Wins: 36
Losses: 2
Draw: 1

Roy Jones
Fights: 48
Wins: 47
Losses: 1
Draws: 0

Marvin Hagler

Fights: 67

Wins: 62

Losses: 3

Draws: 2

Roberto Duran

Fights: 112

Wins: 100

Losses: 12

Draws: 0

Welter-weight

Thomas Hearns

Fights: 61

Wins: 56

Losses: 4

Draws: 1

Lightweight to Light Welter-weight

Oscar Dela Hoya

Fights: 23

Wins: 23

Losses: 0

Draws: 0

Featherweight

Azumah Nelson

Fights: 44

Wins: 39

Losses: 3

Draws: 2

Lightweight

Juilo Caesar Chavez

Fights: 100

Wins: 97

Losses: 2

Draws: 1

data is accurate at the time of writing

Philosophy Quotes of Sifu Marc Davis

 You will achieve clarity of thought when you posses a clear and peaceful mind.

 Learn to be patient and good things will come to you.

 Be positive but not arrogant and you will perform to the best of your abilities.

 One of the highest levels within the martial arts is avoidance not to be there in the first place.

 If you are in a confrontation and can walk away, then do so it takes more strength to walk away.

 In real combat there are no rules, so use everything to your advantage.

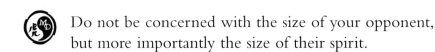 Do not be concerned with the size of your opponent, but more importantly the size of their spirit.

Sparring is simply a very physical game where superior tactics of the mind is the most important thing.

Never give up, the body may be weak but the spirit can overcome anything.

The body is breakable, but your spirit and will can be trained so that nothing and no one can defeat it.

To the unwise, the person who shows kindness and chooses no conflict is weak, don't be fooled.

He who speaks the most often knows nothing.

Never take your opponent for granted, no matter how easy things may seem.

True confidence and security comes from within, nothing and no one can give this to you.

You can never be rid of fear so make it your friend, an ally that you are in complete control of to be used in a positive way.

Always remember there is a time for everything, no matter what the conscience.

If you have negative thoughts about combat don't bother turning up! There is no place for such thoughts.

Always respect life, to show no mercy is to be thuggish and evil. In the end good will over come evil and evil will destroy its self.

Walk with your head high, be the hunter and not the hunted.

If you do not give your opponent anything to use against you, then what can they do.

What we do today will shape our destiny tomorrow.

Strive to be a leader and not a follower.

Anyone can follow but few can lead, remember even when you lead be willing to learn because there is always something.

 Never underestimate anyone in life especially by appearance.

 Do not be concerned with what people think of you, but rather what you think of yourself.

 Always have goodness in your heart, goodness is pure and evil is poluted.

 Time is the master we are simply servants along for the ride.

 Victory is won in the mind and spirit even before the fight has began.

 Look within and beyond to see their fears and insecurities.

 To truly strike your opponent you must go beyond the external and penetrate their very soul.

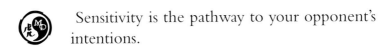 Sensitivity is the pathway to your opponent's intentions.

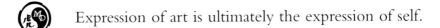 Expression of art is ultimately the expression of self.

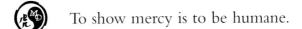 To show mercy is to be humane.

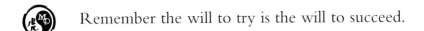 Remember the will to try is the will to succeed.

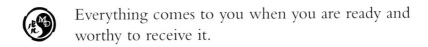 Everything comes to you when you are ready and worthy to receive it.

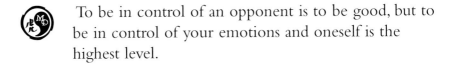 Adaptability is the way of true understanding both in martial arts and life, but always be true to who you are.

To be in control of an opponent is to be good, but to be in control of your emotions and oneself is the highest level.

Attack like the wind and your opponent will not know where your strike is coming from.

The more power you have, then the more responsibilities you have also.

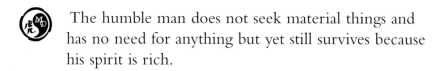 The humble man does not seek material things and has no need for anything but yet still survives because his spirit is rich.

The external is simply an empty vessel, like a car without an engine (pay little attention to it!) The truth and the thing of real importance is what is inside. (The internal.)

The highest level of technique is without thought.

Before you can achieve non-thought you must first learn to think, process and evaluate in a continuous flow.

The journey of martial arts is to explore through exercise, techniques physically, mentally and spiritually to know your self better and ultimately become master of self.

Bruce Lee Philosophy Quotes

Taken from Jeet Kune Do Bruce Lee's commentaries on the martial way, By john Little

Life is something for which there is no answer, it must be understood from moment to moment. The answer we find inevitably conforms to the pattern of what we think we know.

Meditation is freeing your mind from all motives.

The poorer we are inwardly, the more we try to enrich ourselves outwardly.

Only the self-sufficient stand alone, most people follow the crowd and imitate.

In the greater the lesser is, but in the lesser the greater is not.

We live and not live for.

When I listen to my mistakes I have grown.

On cultivating the spirit:

When man comes to a conscious, vital realisation of those great spiritual forces, in science, in business and in life, his progress in the future will be unparalleled.

On cultivating faith in oneself:

Faith too is a state of mind, it can be induced or created by affirmation or repeated instruction to the subconscious mind through the principle of autosuggestion.

It is a well-known fact that one comes to believe whatever one repeats whether true or false. Every man is what he is because of the dominating thoughts, which he permits to occupy his mind.

It is not the obstacle but your reaction to it. (I can if I think I can). .

We are told that talent creates it's own opportunities, but it sometimes seems that intense desire creates not only it's own opportunities, but it's own talents.

Defeat:

Defeat is also a state of mind no one is ever defeated until defeat has been accepted as a reality. To me defeat in anything is merely temporary and its punishment is but an urge for me to greater efforts to achieve my goals. Defeat simply tells me, that something is wrong in my doing it is a path leading to success and truth.

You will never get anymore out of this life than you expect.

No one can hurt you unless you allow him to.

Happiness is good for the body, but sorrow is good for the spirit.

Confuscius Philosophy Quotes

If people have no faith I don't know what they are good for, can a vehicle travel without a link to a source of power.

Exemplary people concern themselves with virtue and small people concern themselves with territory. Exemplary people understand matters of justice and small people understand matters of profit.

Good people inspire others and nurture virtue.

Study without thinking and you are blind, think without study and you are in danger.

The knowing are not confused, the humane are not worried and the brave are not afraid.

Cultivated people reach upward, petty people reach downward.

A Knight who is concerned about a dwelling place is not worthy of being a Knight.

Lao Tze Philosophy Quotes

Taken from Tao Teh Ching

Those who know do not tell, those you tell do not know. Not to set the tongue loose, but to curb it. Not to have edges that catch, but to remain untangled, unblended, unconfused, is to find balance. And he who holds balance beyond sway of love at hate, beyond reach of profit or loss, beyond core of praise or blame, as attained the highest post in the world.

He who knows when he has got enough is rich.

There is no greater calamity than to underestimate your enemy. To do so is to loose your treasure, therefore when opposing troupes meet in battle, victory belongs to the grieving side

He who knows men is clever, he who knows himself has insight, he who conquers men has force he who conquers himself is truly strong.

When a man is living he is soft and supple, when he is dead he becomes hard and rigid. When a plant is living it is soft and tender when it is dead it becomes withered and dry, hence the hard and rigid belong to the company of the dead, the soft and supple belong to the company of the living. Therefore a mighty army tends to fall by it's own weight, just as dry wood is ready or the axe, the mighty and great will be layed low the humble and weak will be exalted.

Existence is infinite, not to be defined.

Those who would take over the Earth and shape it to their will, will never succeed.

I accept destiny is to face life with open eyes.

Yield and you need not break, bend you can straighten, emptied you can hold, torn you can mend.

To yield I have learned is to come back again.

Be utterly humble and you shall hold to the foundation of peace.

He who is open-eyed is open-minded, he who is open-minded is open-hearted, he who is open-hearted is Kingly, he who is Kingly is Godly, he who is Godly is useful, he who is useful is infinite, he who is infinite is immune, he is immune is immortal.

Terminology of Martial Arts

These are some of the most commonly us~~ed~~ terms in both the Chinese and Japanese martial arts

Chinese

Chi gong: Internal energy/power (can be spelt chi gung)

Kung fu: The Chinese form of martial arts, also known as Wu Shu.

Sifu: your instructor, teacher, father

Sijo: the founder of the style/system

Si-Gung: your instructors teacher

Si-Hing: your seniour or older brother

Si Dai: your junior or younger brother

To-Dai: Master of Kung fu

Kwoon: place of training

Chi Sau: sensitivity training

Wu Sau: guard hand

Dan Tien: storage centre for the chi – located just below the navel

Jing: explosive energy

Dim mok: pressure point

Tao: the way, mentally, physically and spiritually

Japanese
Karate: the Japanese form of martial arts

Sensei: instructor

Dojo: place of training

Budo: martial ways

Dan: black belt and above

Deshi: disciple or trainee

Do: the way or path to harmonise body, mind and spirit

Rei: to bow and show respect

Waza: technique

Ukemi: breakfall – how to fall without being hurt

Uchi: strike

Kata: a sequence of movements in a set form

Kumite: sparring competition

Atemi: pressure points

Zanshin: unbroken spirit and a state of total awareness

Glossary

Japanese

Zen discipline that stresses meditation

Karate Do Way of empty hand

Kumite Competition/sparring

Sanshin State of total awareness and oneness

Budo The martial way

Ukemi Break falls

Taisabaki Body shifting

Uke The person who receives the technique being performed

Shite The person who defends

Obi belt

Maitta I surrender

Atemi Pressure points

Ritsu Rei Stand and bow

Za-rei Kneel and bow

Nei Rei Bow to teacher

Chinese

Kwoon Place of training

Dan Tien Where the Chi is located

Dim Mok Vital points/ death touch

Ma Bo Stances/postures

Lap Sau Grabbing hand

Pak Sau Slapping hand

Lan Sau Bar arm

Kwan Sau Double block high and low

Kuo Shu Term used for martial arts of China

Sau Fat Hand techniques

Sifu Master/instructor

Si Gung Instructors teacher

Si Jo The founder of the style of Kung Fu

Si Dai Junior student

Si Bak Senior student

Pak Dar Simultaneous block and attack

Chin Na Joint locking techniques

Tao The way

Thank You

A special thanks for their help with the book to Stephen West, Amy Davis, Richard Reid and Oeystein Ohna.

I would also like to thank my assistant instructors Stuart Gilbert, Dan Lowe, Jonathan Traille, David Jeffery, Gary Nokes for their hard work and dedication, for being their when needed both for me and the MD schools.

References

184

Lee, Bruce. (1997) *Jeet Kune Do* Bruce Lee's Commentaries on th martial way ed. Little, John. Tuttle.

Lee, Bruce. (1997) *The Tao of Gung Fu* A study in the way of chinese martial art ed. Little, John. Tuttle.

Cleary, Thomas (1992) *The Essential Confucius*. The heart of Confucius' teachings in authentic I Ching order. HarperSanFrancisco.

Wu, John, C.H. (1961) *Tao Teh Ching* by Lao Tzu. Shambhala Dragon Editions.